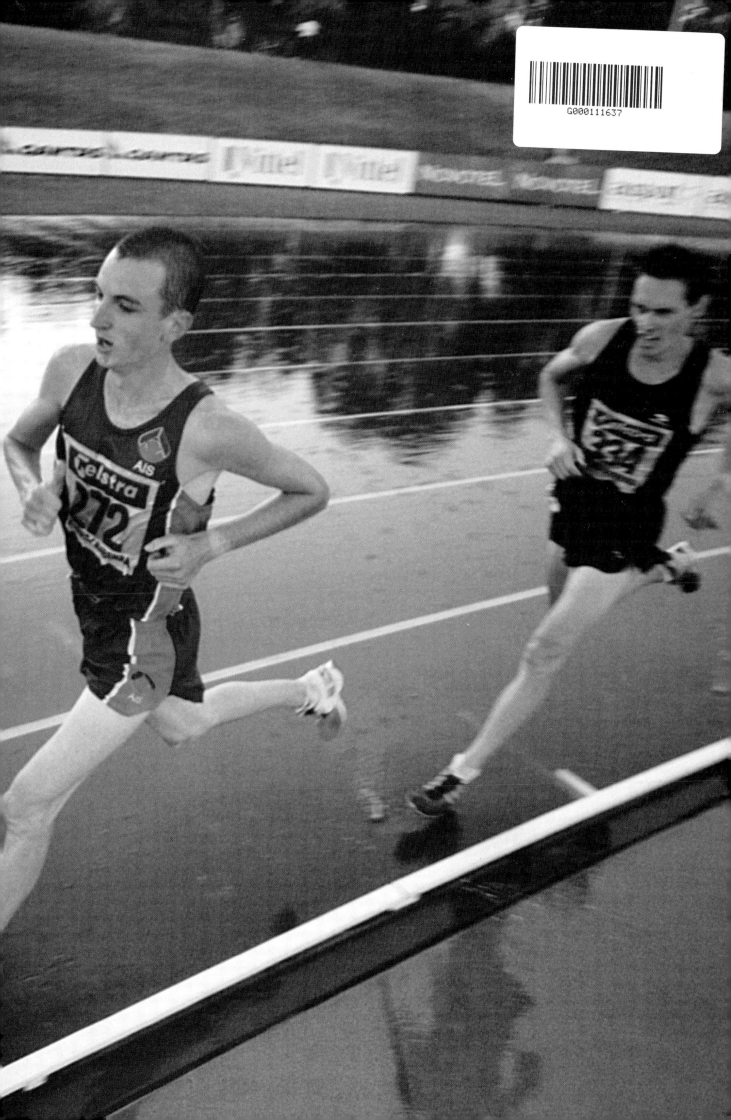

G000111637

The authors would like to thank Katrina Koutoulas, Christina Barca and the FPC Custom Media team for their assistance with *Survival Around the World*. Thanks also to Susan Wright for getting the series off the ground.

We thank the athletes who provided recipes and quotes for this book. Involvement in this project does not imply support of any commercial product or association with the Australian Sports Commission, AIS or Nestlé Australia Ltd.

We are extremely grateful for Alan Hill's assistance in organising the athlete images. Thank you for helping us meet our tight deadline.

Tracy Protas — what would we do without you? Thank you for keeping us on track.

Thanks to our state-based dietitians: Sally Girvan, Deb Kerr, Kerry Leach, Anthony Meade, Sharon Rochester and Nick Wray, and to our tireless athlete trainees: Michael Shelley and Jo-Ann Galbraith.

We also appreciate the assistance of Liz Williams, Lorraine Cullen, Lesley Farthing, Nick Petrunoff and our work experience students: Glenn Kerrins and Andrea Pruscino.

Survival Around the World: A companion book to *Survival from the Fittest* and *Survival for the Fittest* from the athletes of the AIS, has been produced in association with Nestlé Australia Ltd. ABN 77 000 011 316.

First published in 2004 by FPC Custom Media (a division of FPC Magazines).

FPC Magazines is a division of Eastern Suburbs Newspapers Partnership which is owned by General Newspapers Pty Ltd ACN 000 117 322, Double Bay Newspapers Pty Ltd ACN 000 237 598 and Brehmer Fairfax Pty Ltd ACN 008 629 767, 180 Bourke Road, Alexandria, NSW 1435.

Publisher	Naomi Menahem
Production manager	Mark Moes
Concept design	Melissa Mylchreest
Senior designer	Anita Jokovich
Editors	Cate MacKenzie
	Anna Scobie
Food editor/stylist	Jody Vassallo
Photographer	Sue Ferris
Home economists	Chris Sheppard
	Abi Ulgiati
Props stylist	Carlu Seaver

Appliances by Sunbeam. Thanks to Accoutrement, Bayswiss, Bed Bath N' Table, Bison Australia, Cambodia House, Country Road Homewear, David Jones, Design Mode International, Dinosaur Designs, Empire Homewares, Lincraft, Made in Japan, Mud Australia, Myer, No Chintz, Orson & Blake, The Bay Tree, The Essential Ingredient, Village Living, Villeroy & Boch and Wheel&Barrow.

Sports images supplied by the Australian Sports Commission, Australian Institute of Sport, Department of Sports Nutrition and featured athletes. Sports images provided by the Australian Sports Commission/Getty Images on pages: 20, 24, 29, 48, 54, 55, 64, 79, 86, 87, 129, back cover. Images provided by Getty Images on pages: 15, 16 (top left), 17 (bottom left, bottom right), 28 (bottom left), 29 (bottom right), 41, 42 (top left, top right), 43 (top right, bottom left), 53, 54 (top right, bottom right), 64 (top left, bottom left), 65 (top left), 70 (top left, top right, bottom right), 71 (top right, bottom left), 78 (top left, top right, bottom right), 79 (top right, bottom left, bottom right), 85, 86 (top right), 103, 104 (top left), back cover. Images provided by Lonely Planet Images on pages: 27, 28 (top left, top right), 29 (top right, bottom left), 42 (bottom right), 54 (top left), 55 (bottom left), 64 (top right), 65 (bottom left), 71 (bottom right), 86 (top left), 87 (bottom left), 104 (bottom left), 105 (top right, bottom left). Image provided by Photolibrary.com on page 16 (top right).

© 2004 text Australian Sports Commission. For permission to reproduce text, please email copyright@ausport.gov.au
© 2004 food photography and design Nestlé Australia Ltd.

This edition printed by Toppan Printing Co. Hong Kong.

Distributed by Allen & Unwin, 83 Alexander Street, St Leonards NSW 2065.

National Library of Australia Cataloguing-in-Publication Data
Survival around the world.

Includes index.
ISBN 1 74114 383 7.
1. Cookery. 2. Cookery — Health aspects. 3. Athletes — Nutrition. I. Title.
641.5

Nestlé Peters is a trademark owned outside Western Australia by Société de Produits Nestlé SA, a Nestlé company. PETERS is a trademark owned in Western Australia by the Peters and Browne Group, which manufactures and sells ice-cream products in Western Australia. There is no connection between the Nestlé companies and the Peters and Browne Group of Western Australia. The advertised products are manufactured by a Nestlé company and are not available in Western Australia.

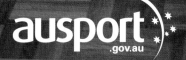

survival

AROUND THE WORLD

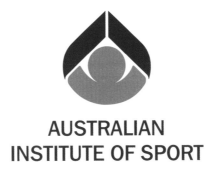

**AUSTRALIAN
INSTITUTE OF SPORT**

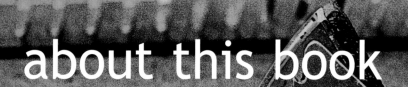

about this book

The life of an elite athlete involves regular travel. When faced with the challenge of eating well in unfamiliar environments, and with limited time and resources, our athletes need recipes that are nutritious, quick, delicious and foolproof. These recipes have been tested in our cooking classes and on the road by athletes, who are tired after training, are trying to juggle many commitments and have limited cooking skills.

To write this cookbook we quizzed our AIS athletes and coaches about their travel wins and mishaps. We have pooled their tips and hints and shared their stories so that others may have successful travel experiences. To extend the information in this book we have developed a website with additional information on travel: www.ais.org.au/nutrition

This cookbook is a great resource for anyone who needs to prepare quick, simple, tasty and nutritious meals — whether you are on the road or at home.

contents

travel tips

Travel is one of the perks of an athletic career but it also provides a range of challenges. These tips will help you achieve your nutritional goals for training and competition while on the move.

top 10 travel challenges:

- Being on the move interrupts your normal training routine and changes your energy needs
- Changing time zones causes jet lag and the need to adjust your eating schedule
- A change in environment, such as sudden exposure to a different altitude or climate, alters nutritional needs and goals
- In a new environment you can experience reduced access to food and food preparation opportunities, compared with the flexibility of being in your own kitchen. Leaving home also means leaving behind important foods and favourite snacks
- The catering plan or team expense account may not stretch to meeting your usual eating habits and nutritional needs, especially snacks and sports foods
- A new food culture and different foods can be overwhelming for young athletes and those with fussy palates
- Hygiene standards with food and water in different countries expose the athlete to the risk of gastrointestinal bugs
- Reading food labels or asking for food may involve tackling a new language
- A substantial part of your new food intake may be coming from hotels, restaurants and takeaway outlets, rather than being tailored to the special needs of athletes
- The excitement and distractions of being away make it easy for young athletes to lose the plot. Common challenges include all-you-can-eat buffets, athlete dining halls, being away from Mum's supervision and being confronted with a whole new array of food temptations.

The following tips will help you to survive, wherever you go. Further information on these strategies can be found in other sections of this book, or on the AIS Department of Sports Nutrition website (www.ais.org.au/nutrition).

1. plan ahead

Good preparation solves many of the challenges of travel. Well before you leave home, sit down and consider the issues you're likely to face on the upcoming trip. Your own past experiences or stories from people who have travelled to this destination will be a good source of information about what to expect, where the challenges will come from and how best to solve them. Things to consider include travel itself, the general food supply at your destination, the specific catering plans that are in place for you, and special nutritional needs arising from your training and competition goals or from the new environment. You will need to follow a good plan while you are away but many elements of this plan will need to be organised ahead of time.

2. eat and drink well while on the move

The challenge starts even before you arrive at your destination. Travel is stressful, changing your nutritional needs (changes in activity levels, increased fluid losses in artificial environments) and opportunities to eat. Changes in time zones also need to be taken into account. A travel eating plan that matches new nutritional goals to food availability will help you arrive at your destination in the best shape possible. For further tips, see 'in transit' (page 8).

3. take a travelling food supply

Once you know about the food supply and catering arrangements on your trip, consider whether foods that are important to your everyday eating are likely to be absent or in short supply at your destination. It is not always necessary to disrupt your familiar and successful eating patterns, or risk missing out on important nutrients. There are a number of foods and special sports products that can travel with you, or ahead of you, to establish a supplementary food supply. Always check with customs/quarantine authorities regarding foods that are restricted from entering certain countries. Travel food supplies may be used to provide snacks as an addition to meals, or to take care of the special needs of competition. For specific tips, see 'travel supplies' (page 9).

4. quickly establish a new routine

Hit the ground running by adjusting your body clock and eating habits to the needs of your destination as soon as possible – even while travelling to get there. Move meal times as quickly as possible to the new time frame. You should factor in the general clock adjustment and the timetable of training and meals that your new environment requires. It may be quite different to the way you do things at home. Remember that you may have different nutritional needs at your destination, due to a change in climate or altitude, or a change in the energy expenditure of your training and competition program. Adjust your meal and snack routine immediately, rather than waiting for problems to occur.

5. be wary of food and water hygiene

Even in 'safe-sounding' destinations, you are exposing yourself to a new set of 'bugs' and new routines of personal and food hygiene. The stress of travel and your new training and competition program may reduce your resistance to illness. Adjust your food and drink choices to minimise your risk of succumbing to gastrointestinal upsets. For tips to guide you in high-risk areas, see 'food safety' (page 10).

6. learn about your new food culture

The fun side of travel is immersing yourself in a new culture. Of course, your priority is to find local ways of achieving your nutritional goals, balancing enough of the tried and true with the adjustments that a new country requires. You will need to identify new foods and eating styles that are compatible with your goals and discover how to tap into the best of what's on offer. For tips on how to identify the issues you might need to consider, see 'approaching different cultures' (page 12).

7. organise catering ahead of time

Whether it be on planes, in hotels or with host families, it pays to let other people know about your catering needs in advance. Special menus and food needs may take time to organise, and in cases where your requests can't be met, advance warning will allow you time to consider alternatives. When travelling in a large group you will be pleased to find that meals are pre-arranged and waiting for you – so the limits of your patience are not tested. For specific tips on how to get organised in advance, see 'eating out' (page 114) and 'self-catering' (page 116).

8. make good choices in restaurants and takeaway outlets

You will need to exercise good judgment when eating in restaurants and takeaway outlets. Important skills to acquire are an understanding of the nutritional characteristics of menu items, and a proactive approach to asking for what you need. For tips on general characteristics of restaurant food, see 'eating out' (page 114). Don't forget to make use of the information about local cuisine provided throughout this book as we travel to the various corners of the world.

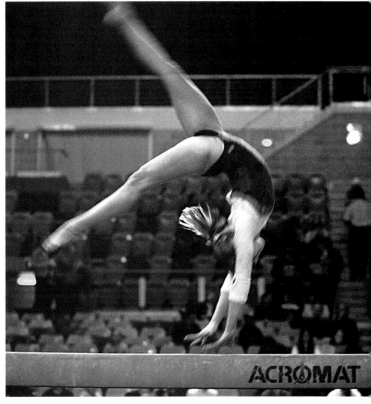

jacqui dunn – gymnast

9. learn smart eating skills for athlete dining halls and all-you-can-eat venues

A new style of eating requires a new style of behaviour. All-you-can-eat and buffet-style eating provide many challenges, even when they are within the confines of an athlete village. For tips on how to ensure that you eat to your plan, rather than succumb to temptations, see 'the athlete dining hall' (page 11).

10. think about the lessons learned for next time

Don't consider the trip to be over until you've had time to debrief. It is important to review what you learned on your travels – what worked, what didn't work, what challenges still need a good solution. Write it all down while it is fresh in your mind because your memories will fade over time. This information will provide an invaluable starting point for preparing for future trips and for sharing your knowledge with others.

in transit

Unusual eating times, inactivity and increased fluid loss during transit can all interfere with performance for the first few days after arriving at your destination. On tours where athletes are constantly on the road, the impact of travelling can become a long-term problem. Whether travelling overseas on a long flight or for just a couple of hours by road or rail, planning and preparation are the keys to successful eating while on the move.

meals and snacks

Excessive consumption of meals and snacks can lead to unwanted body-fat gain. Alternatively, some athletes may find it difficult to meet their nutritional needs while travelling, and weight loss or poor fuel stores could be a risk.

The following strategies can be undertaken to minimise these risks to performance.

1. When flying, contact the airline well in advance of departure to find out if special meals are provided (e.g. low-fat, vegetarian, sports), what they consist of and the timing of the meals during the flight.
2. Plan your food intake in advance and decide which meals you need, and whether your own snacks are also required.
3. On long flights, try to adopt the meal pattern you will have at your destination. This will help to reduce jet lag and adjust your body clock.
4. Forced inactivity when travelling often leads to boredom. To avoid turning to eating to relieve boredom, pack plenty of activities to keep yourself occupied. Reading material, travel games, playing cards, music and audio books can all help to fill in the hours of unaccustomed down time.
5. Athletes with reduced energy needs may not require all the meals and snacks provided during flights. Drinking fluid and chewing sugar-free gum can decrease the temptation to snack excessively. Alternatively, pack your own snacks and decline the in-flight service.
6. When fuel needs are high, pack extra high-carbohydrate snacks to supplement the food provided in-flight.
7. When travelling by road, pack your own supplies, stick to your nutritional plan and avoid being tempted to stop at shops along the way.
8. Pack a supply of snacks in case unexpected delays cause you to miss meals. However, don't be tempted to eat them just because they are there.

Good snack choices when travelling include cereal bars, sports bars, liquid meal supplements, fresh fruit and dried fruit-and-nut mixes. High-fibre snacks can be useful (e.g. wholemeal breakfast bars, dried fruit) if you suffer from constipation on long journeys. It is important to check customs regulations, as you may not be able to take some foods across national or even interstate boundaries.

fluid

The airconditioned environments of trains and buses, and the pressurised cabins in planes cause increased fluid to be lost from the skin and lungs. The risk of becoming dehydrated is high, especially when travel times are long. Symptoms of dehydration can include headaches, fatigue or slight constipation. Although fluid is regularly provided on flights, the small servings are usually insufficient to maintain hydration. When travelling by road or rail, hydration is entirely your responsibility.

Remember to take your own fluids when travelling. Water, sports drinks, juice, soft drinks and tea and coffee are all suitable. Sports drinks provide a small amount of sodium that helps promote thirst (increases the volume of fluid consumed) and decreases urine losses (reduces trips to the toilet). Caffeine-containing fluids such as tea, coffee and cola drinks may cause a small increase in urine production but can still assist with overall fluid balance. Try to drink adequate volumes (for example, 1 cup per hour) to maintain hydration. Avoid alcohol when travelling.

travel supplies

Snacks are an important part of most athletes' eating plans. Whether you are self-catering or relying on others while travelling, it is a good idea to take extra food to supplement your meal arrangements. Depending on the travel destination this may consist of:

▶ favourite foods that are unlikely to be available at the destination
▶ supplies to compensate for poor nutritional quality or unsafe meals
▶ snacks to supplement shortfalls in organised catering
▶ special sports foods or supplements that are a regular part of your nutritional regime or competition preparation.

useful food for travelling

general snacks:

▶ cereal bars
▶ dried fruit-and-nut mixes.

when food availability is limited or food safety is an issue:

▶ dehydrated meals (such as MAGGI 99% Fat Free 2 Minute Noodles, flavoured rice)
▶ canned meals (such as spaghetti, baked beans)
▶ snack packs of fruit
▶ juice concentrate
▶ foil sachets of tuna or salmon
▶ spreads (such as Vegemite, jam, honey)
▶ dried biscuits, crackers or rice cakes
▶ long-life cheese (such as cheese sticks)
▶ powdered liquid meal supplements.

sports foods:

▶ powdered sports drink
▶ powdered liquid meal supplements
▶ sports bars (such as POWERBAR)
▶ gels.

useful equipment for travelling:

▶ single-cup heater to boil water
▶ snap-lock bags or plastic containers
▶ large plastic bowl and cutlery
▶ herbs and spices stored in film canisters to jazz up bland meals.

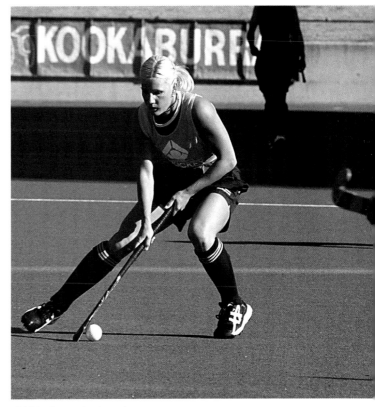

nikki hudson — hockey player

The weight of food supplies needs to be considered, especially when flying. Research the food availability at your destination as thoroughly as possible to avoid taking unnecessary supplies. Pack powdered or concentrated products where possible, such as powdered milk, concentrated juice and dried fruit. Remove any excess packaging from products – snap-lock bags are a good lightweight alternative to tins, jars and boxes. Divide supplies among team members or send a package of supplies ahead to avoid paying for excess baggage. Remember to check with customs/quarantine authorities regarding foods that are restricted from entering certain countries. Check to see if any taxes will be applied.

food safety

The last thing an athlete needs is to get sick before a major competition. Unfortunately, exposure to a new environment can make this a real possibility, especially when food hygiene standards, sanitation and water quality are poor or at a different level to home. There is the risk of food poisoning and water-borne illness everywhere you go, even with local travel. Communal living, the stress of travel and a heavy competition workload can reduce your immunity, therefore increasing your risk. Being aware of the risks and behaving responsibly will improve your chances of an illness-free trip.

water and drinks

It pays to be cautious with water safety. When in doubt about the water supply:

- Use bottled or boiled water for drinking, cleaning teeth and rinsing equipment used for eating or food storage. Boil water for 10 minutes to kill all 'bugs'
- Only consume fluids from containers with unbroken seals or containers that have been opened in your presence
- Wash the external surface of soft drink cans before drinking
- Avoid ice in drinks
- Drinks made from boiled water, such as coffee and tea are usually safe, but added milk may be a source of 'bugs'
- Avoid drinking water from the shower or swimming pools.

food

These tips will help minimise contact with food-poisoning bugs:

- Only eat food that has been cooked, can be peeled or has been washed in safe water
- Food should either be steaming hot or refrigerated. Avoid lukewarm food from bain-maries. Only eat foods that have been thoroughly cooked
- Take care with, and perhaps avoid: fish, pre-prepared salads, soft poached eggs, rare meats, hamburgers, stuffed meats and pastries with cream fillings – these foods are common sources of contamination
- Avoid any fruit with damaged skin. Avoid citrus fruit and melons from street vendors as they may have been injected with water to make them heavier
- Avoid buying food from street vendors. Choose food premises that look clean and busy. Check to see that raw and cooked food is kept separate at all times, cooked food is steaming hot and staff use serving utensils to handle food
- When eating from buffets, ensure chilled food is refrigerated or stored on ice and hot food is kept steaming hot. All dishes should have their own serving utensil and food should be protected from coughs and sneezes by a guard or lid
- Eat food bought from takeaway outlets immediately.

general hygiene

- Always wash your hands before eating or handling food and after going to the toilet or blowing your nose
- When preparing food, to avoid cross-contamination always keep raw foods, such as salads, away from foods that need to be cooked, such as meat
- Use separate chopping boards and cooking utensils for cooked and raw foods.

what to do if you get sick

- See the team doctor if available, otherwise advise the manager or coach
- Drink plenty of fluids, as dehydration is the main danger with diarrhoea
- Take an oral rehydration solution to compensate for lost minerals and salts from severe diarrhoea
- Stick to a bland diet as you recover. You may need to avoid milk, ice-cream and other foods containing lactose, at least in large quantities, for a day or two. This also includes most liquid meal supplements
- Rest, so that you can recover quickly and get back into training
- Think about what food you have eaten in the last two days to determine what may have caused the problem. Avoid the food and warn others about it
- Don't handle or prepare food for others while sick.

the athlete dining hall

Imagine a situation where there is free food, maybe even served 24 hours a day, with numerous choices on offer, plenty of company to enjoy it with, and no sight of Mum to make sure the vegetables are eaten. This is the scenario provided by the athlete villages organised for many of the world's major sporting competitions. As perfect as it sounds, it presents a number of challenges for the travelling athlete. Some of the same challenges are faced when eating in the AIS Dining Hall, all-you-can-eat restaurants and even the buffet-style catering that we recommend because of the flexibility it offers athletic groups. For young and less 'travel savvy' athletes, the temptations and challenges often interfere with achieving nutritional goals. It is important to understand the special challenges of communal eating and to adopt special eating strategies.

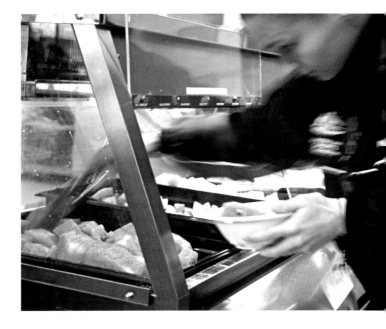

challenges for the athlete

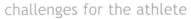

▶ Great quantities of food. You can serve yourself as much as you want from an almost inexhaustible supply. It is easy to eat more than usual and more than you need

▶ Many choices of food all at once. When in doubt, most people have it all. It would be too awful to miss out on something nice

▶ Different and unusual foods. Some people find it difficult to adjust to food that is different to the way they eat at home, or to food that is batch-cooked rather than individually prepared

▶ Lack of supervision. Many young athletes come unstuck when they are first required to take responsibility for their food intake

▶ Distraction. Surrounded by the eating habits of a large group of people, it can be difficult to concentrate on your own nutritional goals. Given the competitive nature of athletes in general, it isn't surprising that official and unofficial eating competitions can take place

▶ Eating for entertainment. Food provides the fuel that powers athletes to gold medals and the achievement of their dreams. But it also fulfils an emotional and social role for athletes and can offer some stress release during the nail-biting weeks of competition. If the dining room becomes a hang-out, a lot of extra food can be demolished in the name of unwinding and relaxing together.

tips for eating well

▶ Clearly know your nutritional goals and how you can choose food to achieve them. If you are unsure or not used to having other people organise meals for you, arrange to see a sports dietitian for some specific advice

▶ Be aware of the total menu on offer and eat to a plan rather than piling a bit of everything on your plate as you move down the food line. Make use of menu boards, or do a lap of the buffet or dining room so that you can plan your meal as you wait in the queue

▶ Convince yourself that piling a bit of everything on your plate is haphazard, unbalanced and usually more than you need – it can quickly lead to unwanted weight gain. But it can also

quickly lead to boredom with the catering, because there is no sense of choosing a different theme each night. Keep things interesting by having a different menu each night

▶ Relax. Remember that there is plenty of food for everyone and menu items will often be repeated. Don't behave as if it is your last meal

▶ Make use of available information, such as nutrition cards, to learn more about the food that is being served. When you are unsure, don't be afraid to ask the waiters or chef

▶ Don't concern yourself with the amount and type of food that other athletes are consuming. The nutritional needs of other athletes may vary quite markedly from your own. Stick to what is right for you

▶ Remove yourself from the food environment once you have finished your meal. Don't expose yourself to boredom eating.

approaching different cultures

Throughout the world, eating is associated with a vast array of customs. Some cultural differences can play havoc with an athlete's usual eating habits. In order to minimise culture shock, consider the following information before leaving home.

typical meal patterns

Don't get caught short by assuming that the evening meal will be the most substantial meal of the day in all countries you visit. Some cultures opt for a large midday meal and a light snack in the evening. If your training or competition schedule causes you to miss a catered lunch, you may need to add some extra snacks to your evening meal. In many countries, breakfast is a much smaller meal than athletes typically require. Be prepared to add your own supplies. In some countries, snacking is not a common practice. This is an important consideration when organising catering or when staying with a host.

timing of meals

In many cultures, it is customary to eat the evening meal quite late, and restaurants tend to have later opening hours than is usual in Australia. This may not suit athletes who need to eat soon after training and grab an early night. Siestas and long lunches are also a feature of many cultures. This can cause all shops to close (usually between 12pm and 2pm). If you are planning to cater for your own lunch, you will need to be organised and shop early.

meal style

Some cultures adopt a shared style of eating, where a variety of dishes are shared among a group. There can be all sorts of cultural norms associated with this, including expectations regarding who serves and who eats first. It is often practice for someone else to serve the guest and provide the best food selection. This sounds good in theory but your host's view of the best foods may differ significantly from your own. For example, in many cultures the fattiest cuts of meat are highly prized.

utensils

Hands, chopsticks, fork and spoon, or knife and fork are all possibilities depending on your travel destination. Most places will cater for westerners and provide a knife and fork. However, it pays to practise eating with the expected utensils before leaving home. When eating with your hands, remember to only use one hand (watch the locals to determine the correct one). When eating a shared meal, it is poor etiquette to use your eating utensils to transfer food to your own plate – always use serving utensils.

grooming

In many cultures it is common practice to wash at the table before eating. Sometimes finger bowls are provided. Alternatively, it may be a damp face washer. When unsure, ask for help or watch those around you before commencing your meal.

dress

In most cultures it pays to be conservative when dressing for group meals. Always change out of your training gear and cover up.

nutrition

It is useful to be familiar with some common foods that are likely to be available at your destination. Investigate the main sources of carbohydrate, fat and protein, and the local varieties of fruit and vegetables. You may need to find substitutes for the foods you count on at home to meet your nutritional needs and to plan for ways to improve the nutritional quality of local meals. It may help to eat at a relevant ethnic restaurant before leaving home to familiarise yourself with possible choices.

language

Language barriers can be one of the most difficult challenges when trying to choose nutritionally appropriate meals in a foreign destination. Try to master some simple phrases and words before leaving home. For example, know how to ask for water, bread and other important items, or to avoid things you hate or are allergic to. Know how to say please, thank you and 'what is … ?'.

how to use this book

The recipes in this book are based on meals that our athletes have eaten or like to eat when they are travelling. As with all of our cookbooks, we have made some modifications so that our recipes:

- Taste delicious
- Are based on nutrient-dense sources of carbohydrate with moderate protein, low fat and high vitamin and mineral levels
- Are quick to prepare and cook
- Use basic techniques
- Use few pots and pans to clean up
- Use ingredients that are easy to find
- Make use of quality convenience products where possible.

Our recipes are suited to those who are just starting out in the kitchen or who have minimal time available for meal preparation. However, we hope to also inspire more skilled cooks who can adapt our recipes to create their own individual taste sensations.

We have provided nutritional information for all our recipes. The nutritional needs of athletes vary considerably. Some, such as endurance athletes, athletes who are growing or athletes aiming to increase muscle mass, have very high fuel needs. Others, such as skill-based athletes and those trying to reduce their body fat levels, require meals that are nutrient-dense but provide less fuel. To better cater for our athletes with lower fuel needs, where possible we have indicated (in coloured type) how to vary the quantity of certain ingredients in some recipes. We have also suggested how to vary the number of serves provided by each meal to cater for athletes with high and lower fuel needs. It is impossible to cater for every athlete and some will find that their individual needs sit somewhere between high and low. It is important to interpret the nutritional information with your own needs in mind.

The following information is provided for each recipe:

ENERGY VALUE
The number of kilojoules in the meal (for calories, divide by 4.2)

CARBOHYDRATE CONTENT
Provided as grams (g) per serve

FAT CONTENT
Provided as grams (g) per serve

PROTEIN CONTENT
Provided as grams (g) per serve.

We have also indicated when recipes are good sources of key nutrients such as iron, calcium and vitamin C.

medals scheme
Our medal scheme helps you quickly assess each recipe and determine how it fits in with your nutrition goals.
- A real winner
- Nearly there
- Needs a little more work

other symbols
✳ Good for freezing

This symbol indicates that the main part of the meal is suitable for freezing (salad ingredients served on the side would not be suitable to freeze). Freeze the whole quantity or, better still, divide it into single serves you can quickly thaw and heat as required. Most meals can be frozen for up to 2-3 months.

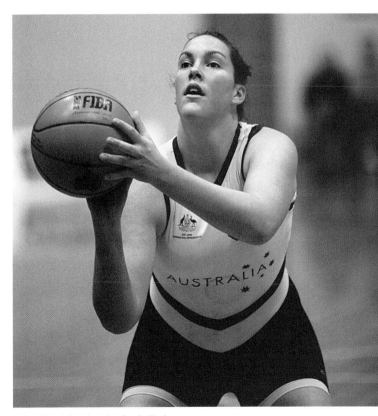

gabrielle richards — basketball player

pacific

Light, flavoursome and easy to prepare tend to be the main criteria for food in the Pacific, whether it is prepared in a kitchen, on a barbecue or in the ground. The abundance of seafood, tender meats and fresh produce means that locals in Australia, New Zealand and the smaller Pacific islands have a healthy diet at their disposal.

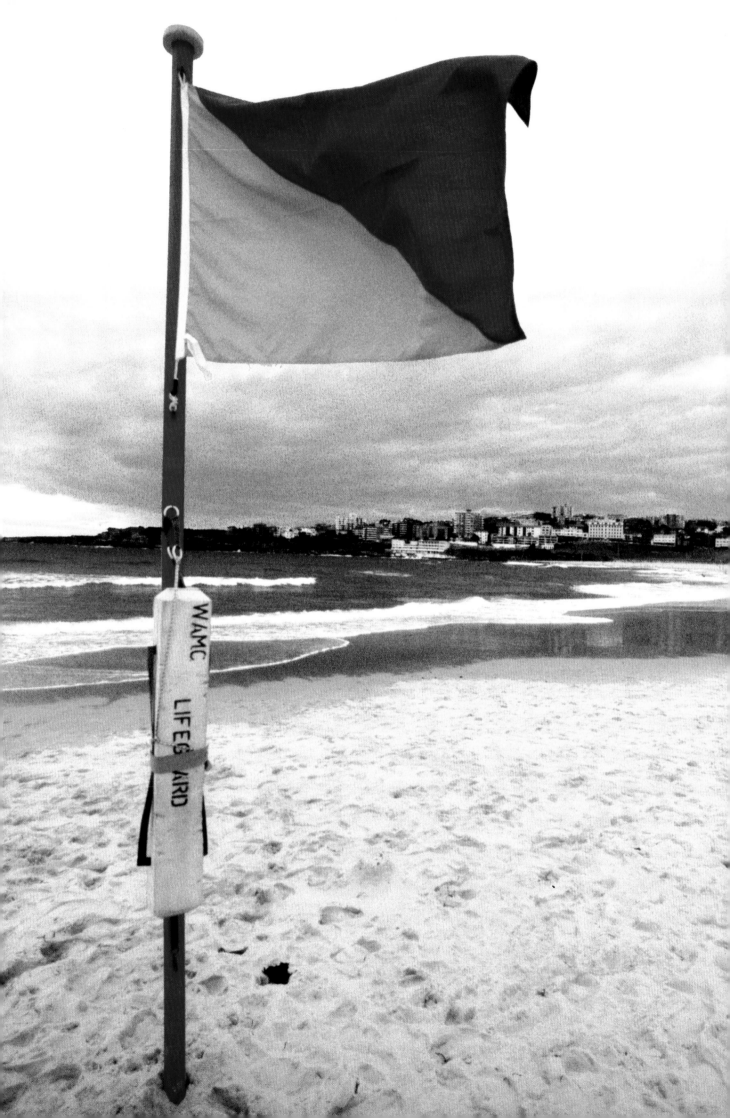

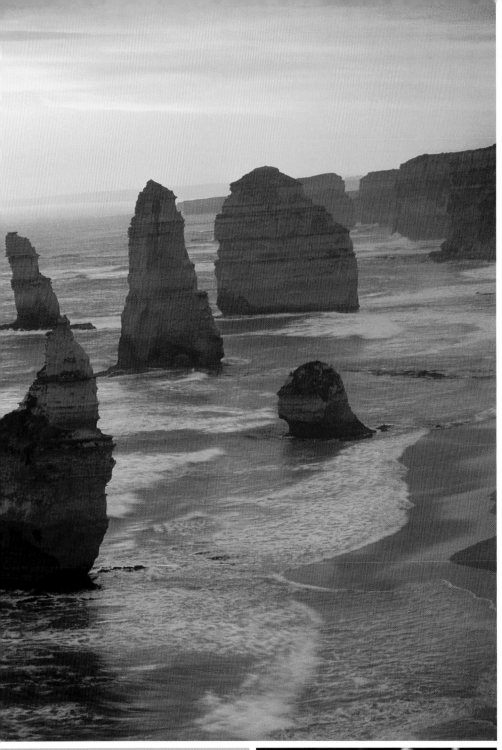

food availability

Larger metropolitan areas offer a wide variety of restaurants, cafés and takeaway outlets, and dining is casual compared with other cultures. Ethnic restaurants, such as Asian, Turkish, Greek and Italian tend to offer the best value. Pubs and clubs often provide good-quality 'counter meals' or buffets but you need to shop around as quality varies. Food courts in large shopping centres can be a quick, economical option for lunch provided you choose carefully. An abundance of quality food and affordable self-catering accommodation make it easy to self-cater in Australia and New Zealand. A limited selection of sports foods, such as sports bars, sports drinks and liquid meal supplements are sold in supermarkets. Specialised products are sold through sports stores. Food availability is limited on some of the smaller islands – take supplies with you.

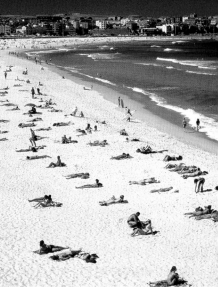

about the culture

Countries within the Pacific region enjoy an eclectic mix of food. In Australia and New Zealand, lasagne, curries, stir-fries and laksa are now as commonplace as traditional favourites, such as roasts. Traditional meals based on fish, poultry, pork, coconut and tropical fruit and vegetables are a feature of many of the Pacific Islands. Australians and New Zealanders typically enjoy three meals a day. Breakfast and lunch are usually small, quick meals and dinner is the main meal of the day. On a population basis, diets tend to be higher in fat and lower in carbohydrate than many athletes require.

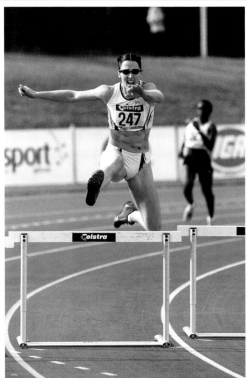

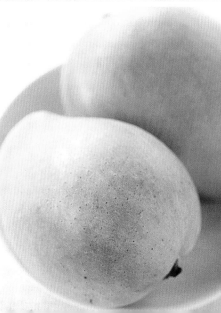

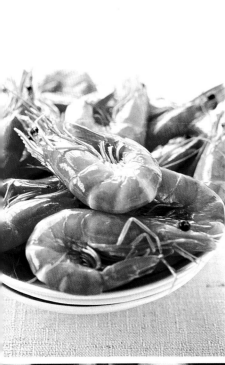

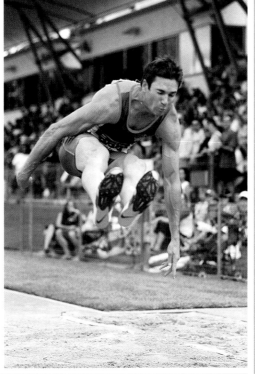

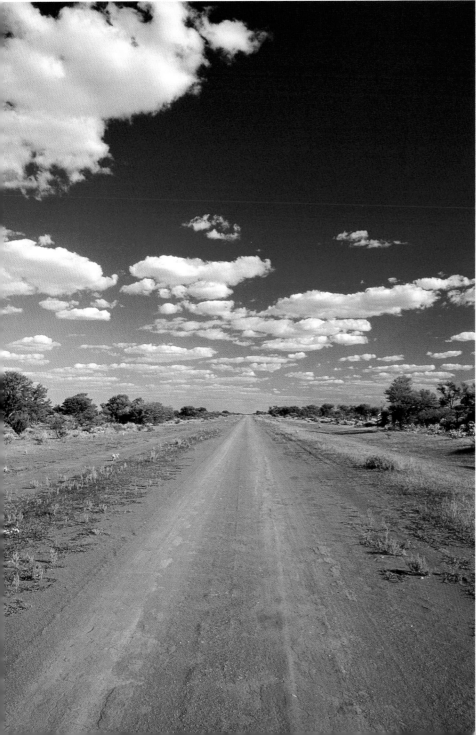

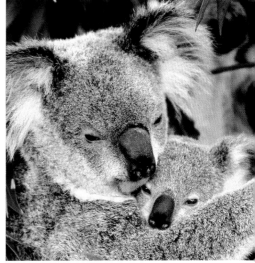

useful tips — perfecting the barbecue

With a few modifications, a barbecue can be a quick, easy and nutritious way to feed a group of hungry athletes:

▶ Choose cuts of meat with minimal visible fat, such as lean rump steak, skinless chicken fillets, trim lamb fillets, kangaroo fillets, fish, burgers made with lean mince and low-fat sausages

▶ Limit meat choices to one or two options. It is tempting to overeat when a large variety is provided. Generally, 100-200g of meat per person is plenty

▶ Use marinades to keep lean meats moist and flavoursome. Seal on one side at a high temperature, reduce the heat, and turn once three-quarters through cooking. Continually poking and prodding the meat will squeeze out all the juices and flavour

▶ Serve a selection of salads, including carbohydrate-based options, such as pasta or rice salad. Use low-fat dressings and herbs to provide flavour. Provide a variety of breads.

main nutrient sources

carbohydrate
Bread, rice, cereal, pasta, noodles, dairy products, fruit and vegetables

protein
Opt for low-fat versions where possible, such as lean meat, skinless poultry, low-fat dairy products and vegetarian sources, such as tofu, lentils and beans

fat
Processed foods are the main source of fat in the diet of Australians and New Zealanders. Read labels before selecting products and be aware of cooking fats when eating out.

pacific

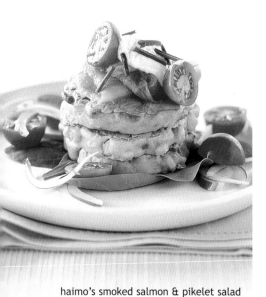

haimo's smoked salmon & pikelet salad

perfect pikelets

▶ Use a non-stick pan on
a low to medium heat —
if it is too hot, the mixture
will brown too quickly and
the centre of the pikelet
will remained uncooked.

▶ If the mixture sticks to the
spoon, lightly spray the
spoon with oil.

▶ Pikelets can be frozen then
reheated in the microwave.

haimo's smoked salmon & pikelet salad   Serves 4-6 *

1 cup self-raising flour
2 eggs
1/2 cup skim milk
1/2 cup chopped fresh coriander
400g can corn kernels,
   rinsed and drained
olive or canola oil spray
150g baby spinach

300g smoked salmon, cut into strips
1 red onion, thinly sliced
1 avocado, sliced
200g cherry tomatoes, halved
200g PETERS FARM Natural
   No Fat Set Yogurt
2 tbs snipped fresh chives
   or chopped dill

Preheat oven to 180°C (350°F). Line a baking tray with non-stick paper. Sift flour into a bowl. Whisk eggs and milk together and pour into dry ingredients, whisk to a smooth batter. Fold in coriander and corn. Lightly spray a large non-stick frypan with oil. To cook 4 pikelets at a time, drop 1 1/2 tablespoonfuls of mixture into pan for each, allowing room for spreading. Cook over medium heat for 3 minutes each side. Transfer to a baking tray and repeat with remaining mixture. Bake pikelets in oven for 10 minutes or until risen. Serve pikelets on a bed of spinach, and top with salmon, onion, avocado and tomatoes. Add a dollop of yogurt and sprinkle with chives or dill.

Analysis	High Fuel	Low Fuel
	4	6
energy (kj)	2245	1497
● protein (g)	34	23
● fat (g)	21	14
● CHO (g)	50	33
● calcium, iron		

fish & chips   Serves 4-6

4-6 large (1kg total) potatoes,
   cut into wedges
1 tbs olive oil
1/2 tsp MAGGI Chicken Stock Powder
1/2 tsp paprika
2 tsp chopped fresh rosemary
600g whiting fillets
200g rocket
2 tomatoes, cut into wedges
1 Lebanese cucumber, cut into chunks
4 rings canned pineapple in natural
   juice, cut into wedges

1/4 cup fat-free dressing
freshly ground black pepper
lemon wedges, to serve
4 large or 6 small bread rolls

dressing:
1 tbs reduced-fat mayonnaise
1 tbs lemon juice
1 tsp grated lemon rind
1 tsp minced chilli
2 tbs finely chopped fresh
   flat-leaf parsley

Preheat oven to 200°C (400°F). Line a baking tray with non-stick paper. Toss potatoes in oil. Combine stock powder, paprika and rosemary and toss through potatoes. Arrange in a single layer on baking tray and bake for 40 minutes or until soft. Meanwhile, to make dressing, combine mayonnaise, lemon juice and rind, chilli and parsley and toss through fish fillets. Cook fish in a non-stick frypan over medium heat for about 2 minutes each side or until golden brown. Combine rocket, tomatoes, cucumber, pineapple, fat-free dressing and pepper to make a salad. Serve with fish, potato chips, lemon wedges and bread rolls.

Tip: Use MAGGI Vegetable Sensations Cajun Wedge Seasoning as a short cut.

Analysis	High Fuel	Low Fuel
	4	6
energy (kj)	2707	1568
● protein (g)	47	29
● fat (g)	12	7
● CHO (g)	79	43
● iron, vitamin C		

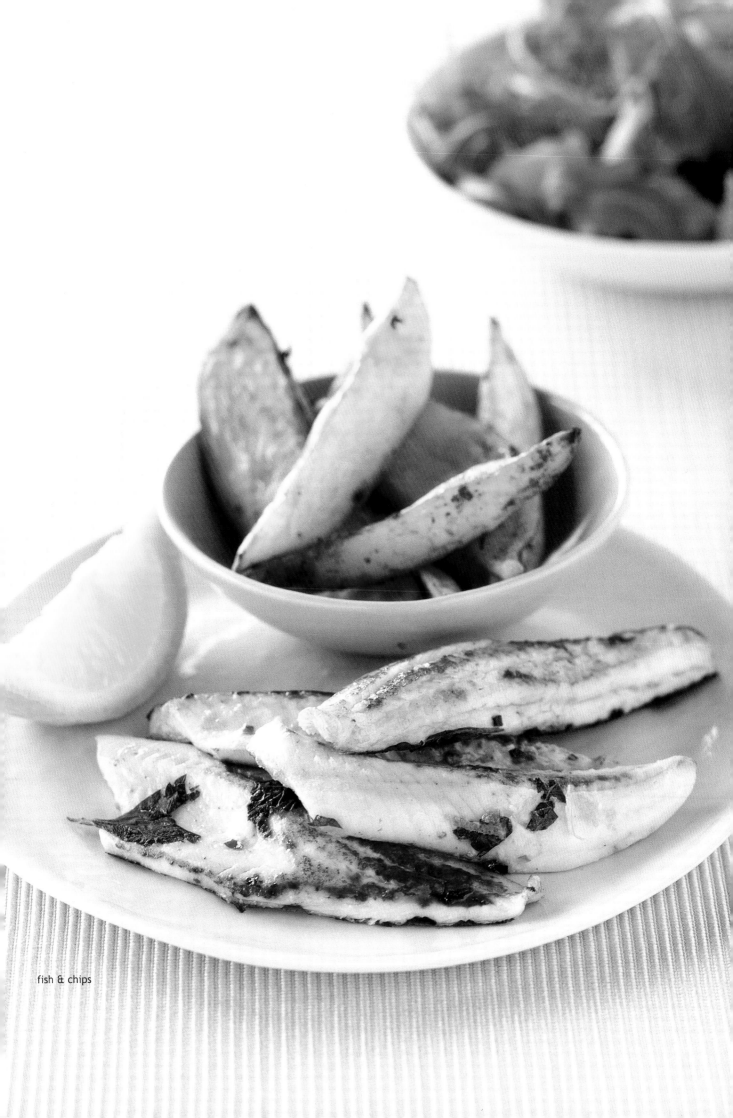

fish & chips

roast lamb & vegies with pumpkin damper   Serves 6-8

800g trim boneless lamb roast
2 cloves garlic, peeled and sliced
3 sprigs fresh rosemary
sea salt and freshly ground black pepper
6-8 desiree potatoes, quartered
500g pumpkin, peeled and deseeded,
    cut into large pieces
6-8 small baby brown onions, peeled
500g baby carrots, tops trimmed
olive or canola oil spray
1 x packet MAGGI Brown Onion
    Gravy Mix
1 tbs mint jelly

pumpkin damper (omit for Low Fuel):
2¹/2 cups self-raising flour
1 tsp baking powder
1 tsp salt
¹/4 cup grated parmesan cheese
2 tbs chopped fresh herbs (such as
    parsley, thyme and rosemary)
1 egg
1 cup cooked mashed (approx 400g
    uncooked) pumpkin
30g butter or margarine, melted
¹/4 cup skim milk

Preheat oven to 200°C (400°F). Place lamb on a rack in a baking dish. Make small incisions in top of lamb and fill with garlic and rosemary. Sprinkle with salt and pepper. Bake for 40 minutes for medium-rare or until cooked to your liking. When lamb has been cooking for 15 minutes, place vegetables in a large baking tray, lightly spray with oil and add to the oven. Bake vegetables for 40 minutes or until golden and tender, turning a few times during cooking. When lamb is cooked, transfer to a plate and cover loosely with foil. Allow to rest for 15 minutes before carving. Meanwhile, combine gravy mix, mint jelly and 1 cup hot water in a small saucepan and cook, stirring, over medium heat until gravy boils and thickens. Serve lamb with potatoes, pumpkin, onions, carrots and gravy. To make damper (omit for Low Fuel), sift flour and baking powder into a bowl. Stir in salt, parmesan and herbs. Whisk together egg, pumpkin, butter or margarine, and milk and add to dry ingredients. Mix to form a soft dough. Turn onto a lightly floured surface and knead until smooth. Place on a baking tray lined with non-stick paper, then score into 6-8 portions using a flat-bladed knife. Bake at 200°C (400°F) for 25 minutes or until cooked.

Analysis	High Fuel 6	Low Fuel 8 no damper
energy (kj)	2846	1752
protein (g)	46	37
fat (g)	16	9
CHO (g)	81	42
calcium, iron, vitamin C		

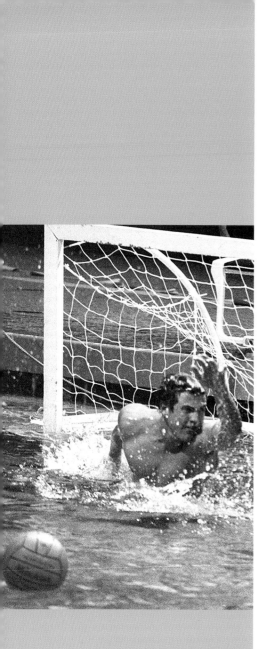

**luke quinlivan —
water polo**

"For a quick meal on the road, I make a risotto-style dish. I take some arborio rice and stock, then throw in whatever meat, vegetables and seasonings I have on hand. It's a really versatile meal and much more exciting than pasta."

warm kangaroo salad   Serves 4-6

1-2 tsp minced garlic
¹/4 cup balsamic vinegar
1 tbs olive oil
1 tsp blueberry jam
500g kangaroo fillets
500g pumpkin, deseeded, cut into
    1cm-thick slices
200g green beans, cut into 5cm lengths
200g broccolini, woody ends trimmed
200g baby spinach

¹/4 cup fresh flat-leaf parsley leaves
³/4 cup fresh blueberries
4 large or 6 small bread rolls

dressing:
1 tbs olive oil
2 tbs balsamic vinegar
1 tsp minced chilli
freshly ground black pepper

Combine garlic, vinegar, oil, jam and kangaroo in a bowl. Set aside for 15-30 minutes to marinate. To make dressing, combine ingredients; set aside. Preheat oven to 200°C (400°F). Place pumpkin on a baking tray lined with non-stick paper and bake for 15 minutes or until tender. Cook kangaroo in a non-stick frypan over medium-high heat for 5-8 minutes each side or until browned and tender. Remove from heat and allow to rest for 5 minutes. Blanch beans and broccolini in boiling water for 1 minute. Slice kangaroo into 1cm-thick strips. Divide beans, broccolini, spinach and parsley among plates. Top with pumpkin and kangaroo. Drizzle with dressing, sprinkle with blueberries and serve with bread rolls.

Analysis	High Fuel 4	Low Fuel 6
energy (kj)	2245	1505
protein (g)	42	28
fat (g)	15	10
CHO (g)	52	35
iron, vitamin C		

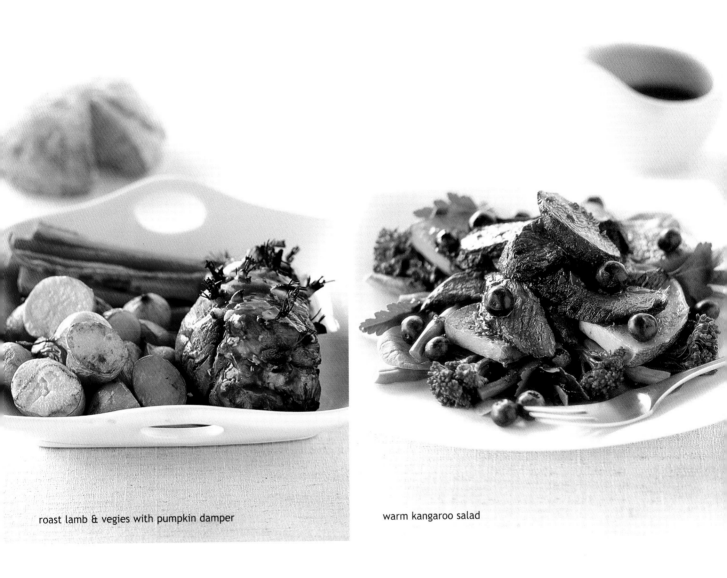

roast lamb & vegies with pumpkin damper

warm kangaroo salad

"Whenever I travel within Australia, I always pack my Chinese essential — soy sauce flavoured with hot chillies. I add it to everything to create some real Chinese flavour!"

— tian ju ping, AIS gymnastics coach

prawn & vegetable skewers   Serves 4-6

You will need 12-16 **bamboo skewers,
  soaked in water**
1 1/2-2 cups rice
800g large green king prawns, peeled
  and deveined, tails intact
1/4 cup each MAGGI Sweet Chilli Sauce
  and MAGGI Chilli & Garlic Sauce
1/4 cup soy sauce

1 red capsicum, deseeded
  and cut into chunks
2 zucchini, cut into chunks
6-8 button mushrooms, halved
1/2 cup canned pineapple pieces
  in natural juice, drained
16 cherry tomatoes

Cook rice according to packet instructions. Preheat barbecue grill plate to medium-high heat.
Rinse prawns and place in a bowl with sauces. Set aside for 10-15 minutes to marinate.

Analysis	High Fuel	Low Fuel
	4	6
energy (kj)	2621	1746
protein (g)	51	34
fat (g)	3	2
CHO (g)	94	63
calcium, iron, vitamin C		

Alternately thread capsicum, zucchini, mushrooms,
pineapple and tomatoes onto skewers. Thread prawns onto
separate skewers, fitting 3-4 prawns on each skewer. Place
vegetable skewers on grill plate and cook for 3-5 minutes,
turning occasionally. Add prawn skewers and cook for a
further 3-5 minutes, turning occasionally. Serve with rice.

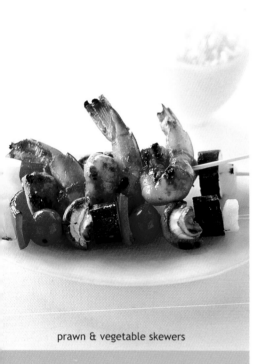

prawn & vegetable skewers

perfect prawns

▶ If you would like to wash
  prawns before cooking,
  use salty water as fresh
  water will remove their
  naturally salty flavour.
▶ Prawn heads and shells
  are ideal to use when
  making stock. However,
  if discarding them, store
  in the freezer until rubbish
  day to avoid nasty odours.

pumpkin & bean burgers   Makes 6 ✳

1 cup finely diced pumpkin
olive or canola oil spray
1 onion, finely chopped
1 tsp minced garlic
1 tsp minced chilli
1-2 tbs curry powder
2 x 400g cans butter beans,
  rinsed and drained
200g frozen spinach, defrosted and
  excess water squeezed out

1/2 cup couscous
1/4 cup chopped fresh flat-leaf parsley
2 tbs chopped fresh chives
12 slices sourdough bread
1 cup low-fat beetroot dip
100g mixed lettuce leaves
3 tomatoes, sliced
1 cup chutney

Cook pumpkin in microwave on HIGH for 1-2 minutes or until soft, drain. Spray a non-stick
frypan with oil and cook onion, garlic and chilli over medium heat until soft. Add curry powder
and cook for 1 minute. Mash beans and pumpkin and combine with spinach, couscous, herbs

Analysis	High Fuel	Low Fuel
	2 burgers	1 burger
energy (kj)	2860	1430
protein (g)	28	14
fat (g)	8	4
CHO (g)	118	59
calcium, iron, vitamin C		

and onion mixture. Wet hands and shape mixture into 6 flat
patties. Refrigerate for 15 minutes. Preheat barbecue to
medium heat and cook patties for 5 minutes each side or
until heated through. Spread 6 slices of sourdough with
beetroot dip. Top with lettuce and tomatoes, then a patty, a
spoonful of chutney and another slice of bread.

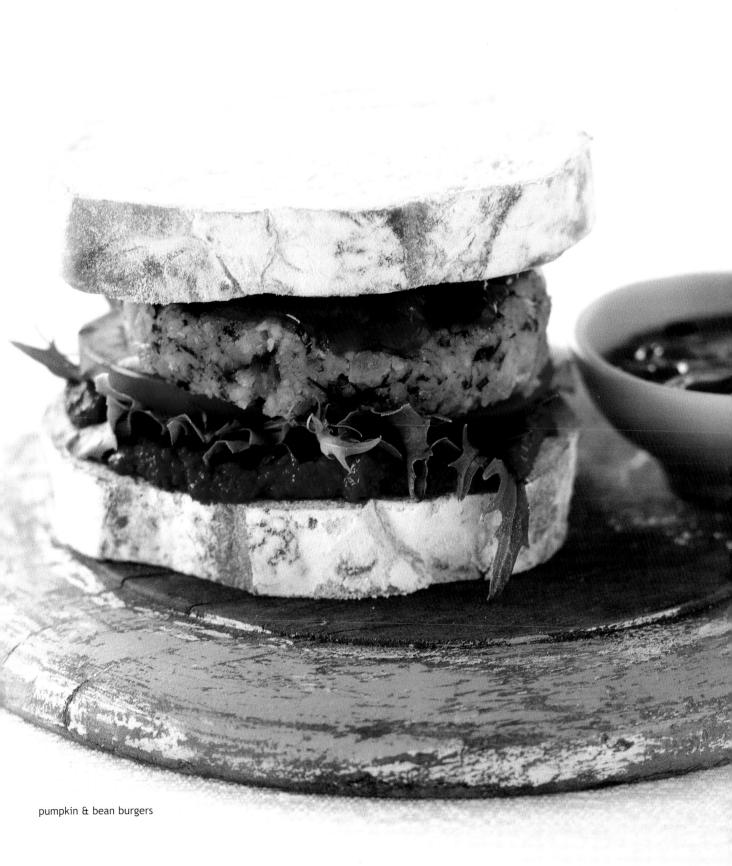

pumpkin & bean burgers

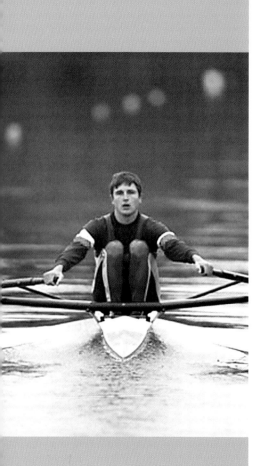

fruity anzac slice and MILO milkshake Makes 16 slices

1¹/2 cups rolled oats
1¹/2 cups cornflakes
¹/3 cup desiccated coconut
80g dried apricots, diced
80g dried pears, diced
395g can NESTLÉ Sweetened
  Condensed Skim Milk
¹/4 cup brown sugar

MILO milkshake (Serves 2):
2 cups reduced-fat milk
1 banana, roughly chopped
2 tbs PETERS FARM Natural
  No Fat Set Yogurt
¹/2 cup MILO powder, plus extra
  to sprinkle
Ice cubes

Anzac Slice	
Analysis	Per slice
energy (kj)	642
protein (g)	4
● fat (g)	2
● CHO (g)	30

MILO Milkshake	
Analysis	2 serves
energy (kj)	1098
● protein (g)	15
● fat (g)	6
● CHO (g)	38
● calcium, iron, vitamin C	

Preheat oven to 180°C (350°F). Line an 18cm x 28cm slice tray with non-stick paper. Combine oats, cornflakes, coconut and dried fruit in a large bowl. Combine condensed milk and sugar in a microwave-safe bowl and heat in microwave on MEDIUM for 5 minutes, stirring after each minute, until thick and pale brown. Add to dry ingredients and mix until thoroughly combined. Press mixture into tray using a spoon dipped in hot water. Dip a knife in hot water and score slice into 16 fingers. Bake for 20-30 minutes or until firm. Leave to cool in tray before slicing into fingers with a serrated knife. To make MILO Milkshake, process all ingredients in a blender until thick and creamy. Pour into glasses and sprinkle with extra MILO powder.

baked nectarines with anzac crumble Serves 4-6

6 large nectarines, halved,
  stones removed
6 Anzac biscuits, crushed
2 tbs honey

1 tsp ground cinnamon
1 tsp vanilla essence
4 x 200g tubs NESTLÉ All Natural
  99% Fat Free Vanilla Yogurt

Analysis	High Fuel	Low Fuel
	4	6
energy (kj)	1470	980
protein (g)	12	8
● fat (g)	7	4
● CHO (g)	62	41
● calcium		

Preheat oven to 180°C (350°F). Place nectarine halves, skin-side down, in an ovenproof dish. Combine biscuits and honey; place a little in the hollow of each nectarine. Add cinnamon and vanilla essence to 1 cup water and pour into base of dish. Bake for 20 minutes or until nectarines are soft. Remove from dish and serve with yogurt.
Tip: Use apples if nectarines are not available.

haimish karrasch — lightweight rower

"I enjoy coming home to Australian food, especially because I can cook it myself. We travel for three months of the year, and I get sick of hotels and restaurants and having other people decide what's on the menu. I love fresh, light and healthy foods and these were the basis of the salmon & pikelet salad recipe I developed for this book [see recipe, page 18]. One day, I'd like to settle down and buy a restaurant, and be my own chef!"

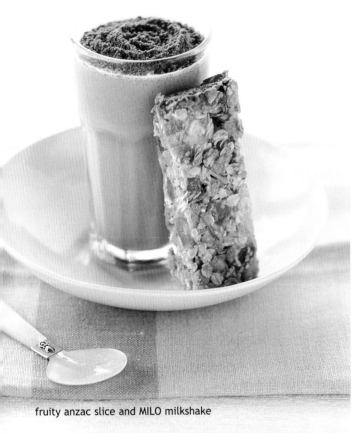

fruity anzac slice and MILO milkshake

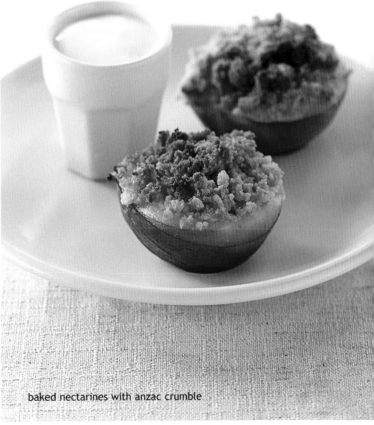

baked nectarines with anzac crumble

"I spend six months of the year overseas, so I have had to learn to fend for myself. I'm not known for my culinary skills, so I often have to go out for my evening meal. I'm hoping *Survival Around the World* will help improve my cooking skills."

— brad kahlefeldt, triathlete

north.
america

Although the cuisine available here is as varied as its broad cultural mix, North America has developed a unique assortment of sweet and savoury dishes to call its own. As well as teaching the world how to prepare turkey every which way, North America is known for muffins, bagels, cheesecake, cookies and flavoured coffees.

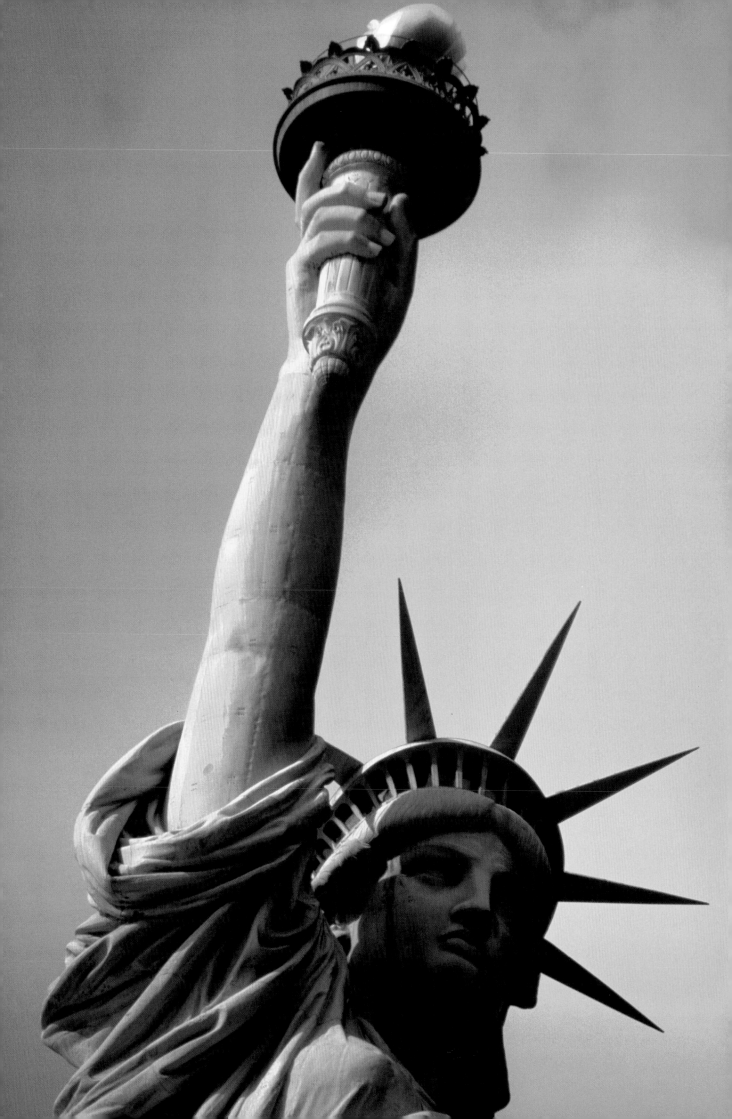

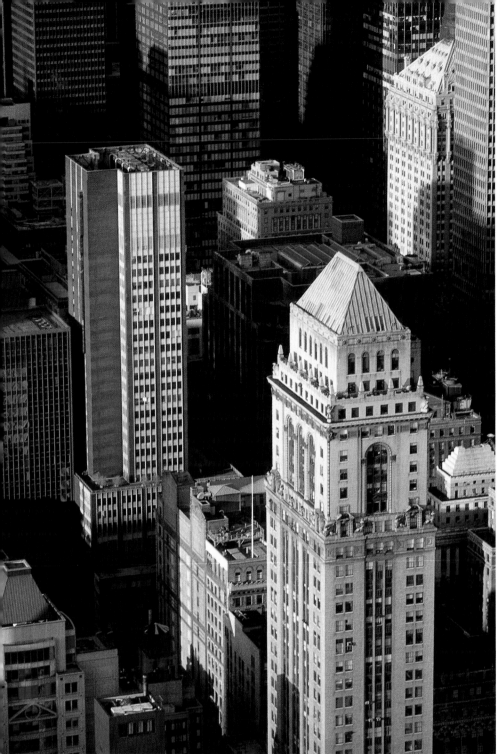

food availability

You will find everything you need for self-catering in North America, plus a whole lot more. Making sense of the numerous processed foods can be a challenge. Many breakfast cereals are loaded with sugar – look for Weetabix, Quaker Oats, Grape Nuts and Raisin Bran or visit the local health store. There is usually an excellent assortment of frozen/fresh pizzas in supermarkets – you can add extra toppings, such as sliced tomato, capsicum and mushrooms to increase your vegetable intake. Some great snack choices include:

▶ Fig Newtons (fruit-filled biscuits)
▶ Bagels (try blueberry)
▶ Low-fat crisps (try Baked Lays)
▶ Baked corn chips (low-fat version of corn chips) with salsa
▶ Flavoured rice cakes – regular or bite sized (try Caramel Corn).

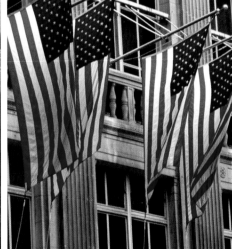

about the culture

North American cuisine is renowned for its focus on protein-rich foods, with beef taking centre stage. It is easy to overeat in the US, as it is commonly perceived that 'bigger equals better'. Fast-food outlets are prolific throughout North America and eating on the run is common practice. You'll have a variety of food choices at your fingertips, but the healthier options are mostly off the beaten track so it's best to research your destination before you go.

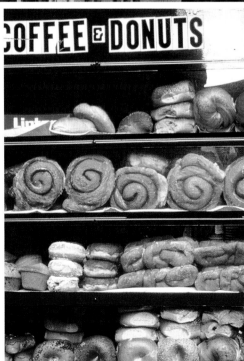

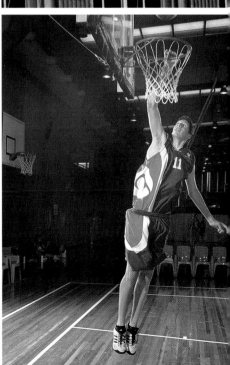

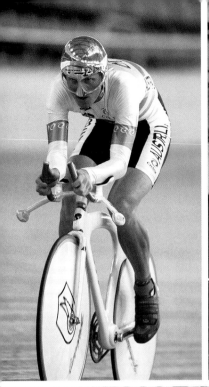
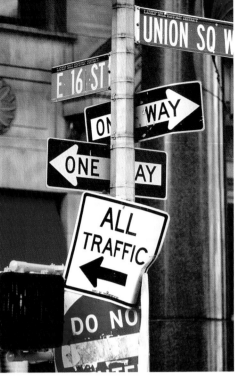

useful tips —
eating out in the usa

- Ask for smaller serves, avoid combination dishes (such as chicken *and* prawns) that double up on quantities, or be prepared to leave food on your plate. Try ordering one main meal (entrée) between two people, and add extra salad and vegetables to balance the meal
- Be wary of 'upsizing'. For only a few extra dollars you can wreak havoc on your dietary goals.
- Hotel breakfasts often consist of an assortment of high-fat donuts and pastries. Be prepared to resist them by travelling with your own cereal and long-life milk supply
- Crisps are served regularly at cafés, sandwich bars and other eating establishments with a sandwich or bagel. Ask for the reduced-fat variety or go without
- Many meals are accompanied by high-fat options such as fries, wedges, okra and onion rings. Despite being a source of carbohydrate, these can significantly increase your daily fat and kilojoule intake
- Americans have a tendency to drown salads in high-fat dressings. Ask about the dressing before opting for a salad
- Mexican restaurants provide free corn chips and salsa as soon as you are seated. Combine this with endless refills of soft drink (pop) and it is easy to be full before your meal arrives
- Bagels are an excellent choice for a snack, lunch or breakfast. They are often served with cream cheese, so make sure you ask for low fat.

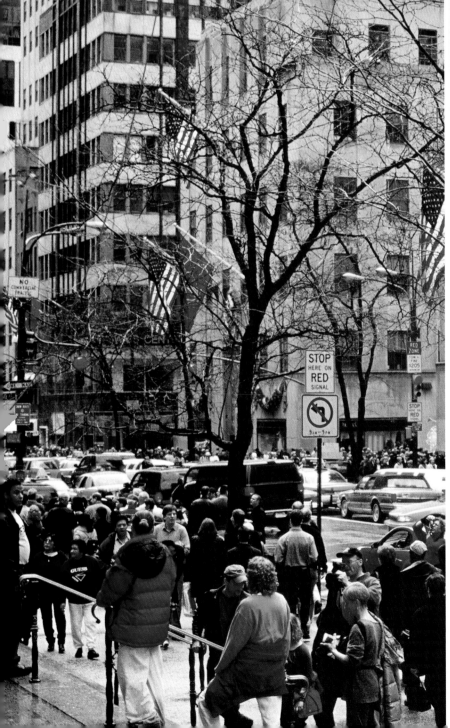

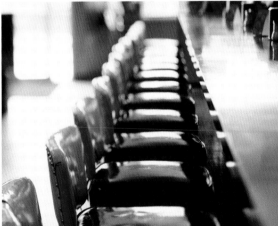

main nutrient sources

carbohydrate
A variety of sources, but beware of added fats

protein
Servings of protein foods are usually large

fat
'Fat free' foods are abundant in North America, but be careful as 'fat free' does not mean kilojoule free.

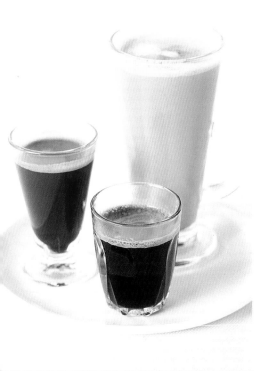

the perfect blend

The majority of North America seems to wake up to freshly brewed coffee — the only trouble is deciding on your favourite blend. Whether you prefer the bitterness of an espresso, the milkiness of a latte or the sweetness of a flavoured coffee, there are three rules to adhere to: make sure the water you use is good enough to drink, always warm your coffee cup and never reheat.

banana & white choc muffins   Makes 12 ☀

1¹/₂ cups self-raising flour
1 cup wholemeal self-raising flour
³/₄ cup brown sugar
¹/₂ cup NESTLÉ White Choc Bits
1 tbs margarine, melted

1 cup skim milk
1 egg
1 tsp vanilla essence
2 ripe bananas, well mashed

Preheat oven to 180°C (350°F). Line a 12-hole muffin pan with paper muffin cases. Sift flours into a large bowl, then add husks. Stir in sugar and choc bits and make a well in the centre. In a small bowl, use a fork to whisk together margarine, milk, egg, vanilla essence and bananas, then add to flour mixture. Stir gently until mixture is just combined (do not over-beat). Spoon mixture into cases. Bake for 20-25 minutes or until muffins are well risen and spring back to the touch. Leave in pan for a few minutes, then transfer to a wire rack to cool.

Analysis	Per muffin
energy (kj)	887
protein (g)	5
fat (g)	4
CHO (g)	38

variations:

chocolate raspberry muffins

Use 2¹/₂ cups self-raising flour and omit wholemeal flour. Sift ¹/₄ cup NESTLÉ baking cocoa and ¹/₂ teaspoon bicarbonate of soda with flour. Use caster sugar instead of brown sugar and NESTLÉ Dark Choc Bits instead of White Choc Bits. Omit vanilla essence and bananas. Fold 300g frozen raspberries through mixture before spooning into muffin cases.

Analysis	Per muffin
energy (kj)	946
protein (g)	5
fat (g)	4
CHO (g)	41

lemon coconut muffins

Use 2¹/₂ cups self-raising flour and omit wholemeal flour. Use caster sugar instead of brown sugar. Stir in ¹/₂ cup desiccated coconut and grated rind of 1 lemon with sugar. Omit NESTLÉ White Choc Bits, vanilla essence and bananas. Add 100ml lemon juice to egg mixture. Half-fill muffin cases with mixture, then add 1 teaspoon lemon butter to each. Top with remaining mixture. Make a small well in top of each and add an extra ¹/₂ teaspoon lemon butter.

Analysis	Per muffin
energy (kj)	888
protein (g)	5
fat (g)	3
CHO (g)	41

pumpkin & cinnamon muffins

Use 2¹/₂ cups self-raising flour and omit wholemeal flour. Sift 2 teaspoons ground cinnamon and 1 teaspoon ground nutmeg with flour. Reduce brown sugar to ¹/₃ cup. Omit NESTLÉ White Choc Bits and vanilla essence. Replace bananas with ³/₄ cup cooked mashed pumpkin and ¹/₄ cup prune puree. Combine 3 tablespoons chopped walnuts and 2 tablespoons extra brown sugar and sprinkle on top of muffins before baking.

Analysis	Per muffin
energy (kj)	727
protein (g)	5
fat (g)	4
CHO (g)	30

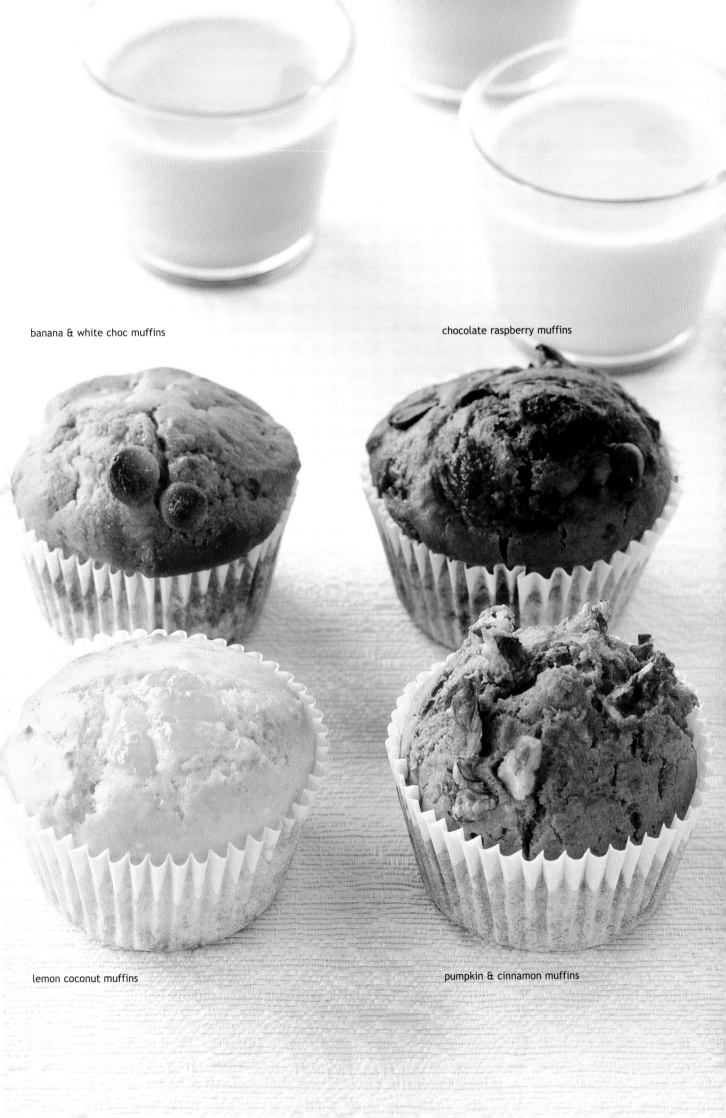

banana & white choc muffins

chocolate raspberry muffins

lemon coconut muffins

pumpkin & cinnamon muffins

roast beef bagel Serves 1

1/2-1 bagel, split
1 tbs horseradish
2 slices roast beef

3 thin slices cucumber
3 slices tomato
small handful cress

Analysis	High Fuel 1 bagel	Low Fuel open bagel
energy (kj)	1816	1262
protein (g)	34	29
fat (g)	8	7
CHO (g)	55	30
iron, vitamin C		

Spread base of bagel with horseradish. Top with remaining ingredients. For High Fuel, top with second bagel half. For Low Fuel, leave as an open bagel.

cream cheese & vegie bagel Serves 1

1/2-1 bagel, split
1 tbs low-fat spreadable cream cheese
1 lettuce leaf, torn
1/2 small carrot, grated

3 slices tomato
1 egg, hard-boiled
freshly ground black pepper

Analysis	High Fuel 1 bagel	Low Fuel open bagel
energy (kj)	1744	1190
protein (g)	20	16
fat (g)	12	11
CHO (g)	55	30
calcium		

Spread base of bagel with cream cheese. Top with remaining ingredients. For High Fuel, top with second bagel half. For Low Fuel, leave as an open bagel.

passion power Serves 1

65g POWERBAR Protein Plus
   Chocolate Powder*
200ml skim milk

2 tbs passionfruit pulp
2 scoops PETERS Light & Creamy
   Ice-Cream

Analysis	1
energy (kj)	1652
protein (g)	26
fat (g)	4
CHO (g)	64
calcium, iron, vitamin C	

Process chocolate powder, skim milk, passionfruit pulp and ice-cream in a blender until smooth.
* Available from selected supermarkets and sports stores.

barney's blended juice Serves 1-2

1 cup pineapple juice
1 banana
6 strawberries, hulled

200g tub NESTLÉ All Natural
   99% Fat Free Vanilla Yogurt

Analysis	High Fuel 1	Low Fuel 2
energy (kj)	1808	904
protein (g)	14	7
fat (g)	4	2
CHO (g)	84	42
calcium, vitamin C		

Process pineapple juice, banana, strawberries and yogurt in a blender until smooth.
Tip: For an icy cold option, use a frozen banana.

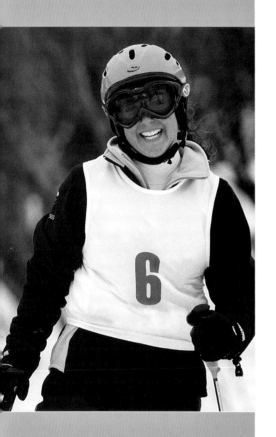

manuela berchtold — freestyle skier

"I have spent many seasons based at Steamboat Springs, Colorado, USA. The family I always live with introduced me to this fantastic soup, which I call Steamboat Springs Soup [see recipe, page 34]. I have been making it on tour ever since first tasting it. I've modified it a bit to lower the fat content. It fills me up without the heavy feeling that some meals can give me."

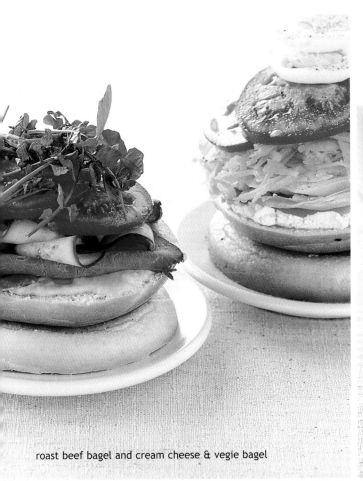

roast beef bagel and cream cheese & vegie bagel

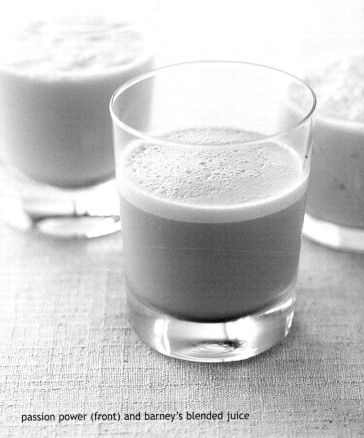

passion power (front) and barney's blended juice

"Last time I was in the States, it took me a while to work out that when people ask if you want cream in your tea or coffee, they actually mean milk."

— jeff dowdell, basketball player

fish chowder Serves 4-6 *

olive or canola oil spray
1 large onion, diced
2 slices ham, diced
2 celery sticks, diced
1 carrot, diced
1 tsp minced garlic
2 tbs plain flour
3 large (600g total) potatoes,
    peeled and chopped
2 cups fish or vegetable stock

375ml can CARNATION Light
    & Creamy Evaporated Milk
1 tbs lemon juice
500g white fish fillets (such as
    flathead, whiting), cut into chunks
300g can corn kernels,
    rinsed and drained
2 tbs snipped fresh chives
4 large or 6 small bread rolls

Spray a non-stick saucepan with oil and cook onion, ham, celery, carrot and garlic over medium heat for 5 minutes or until soft. Add flour and potatoes and cook, stirring, for 1 minute. Add stock, evaporated milk and lemon juice, reduce heat to low and simmer for 10-15 minutes or until potatoes are soft. Add fish and corn. Cook, stirring, over medium heat for 5 minutes or until fish is cooked through. Ladle soup into bowls and garnish with chives. Serve with bread rolls.

Analysis	High Fuel	Low Fuel
	4	6
energy (kj)	2828	1650
● protein (g)	52	32
● fat (g)	9	5
● CHO (g)	91	51
● calcium, iron, vitamin C		

steamboat springs soup Serves 4-6 *

olive or canola oil spray
1 onion, diced
1 tsp minced garlic
1 tsp minced chilli
500g chicken breast fillets, chopped
1 tsp chilli powder
2 tsp ground cumin
1 tsp dried oregano
1 litre MAGGI Real Chicken Stock

400g can diced tomatoes
4 flour tortillas
2 tbs chopped fresh coriander,
    plus extra to garnish
400g can corn kernels,
    rinsed and drained
1/4 cup grated low-fat cheese
4 large or 6 small bread rolls

Spray a non-stick saucepan with oil and cook onion, garlic and chilli over medium heat until soft. Add chicken and cook until browned all over. Add chilli powder, cumin and oregano and cook for 1 minute. Add stock and tomatoes, then reduce heat to low and simmer for 10 minutes or until chicken is tender. Meanwhile, preheat grill to medium-high heat and toast tortillas until crisp. Break into pieces. Add coriander to soup and simmer for 5 minutes. Stir corn through, then ladle soup into bowls and top with tortillas, cheese and extra coriander. Serve with bread rolls.

Analysis	High Fuel	Low Fuel
	4	6
energy (kj)	2534	1453
● protein (g)	45	28
● fat (g)	14	9
● CHO (g)	70	37
● iron		

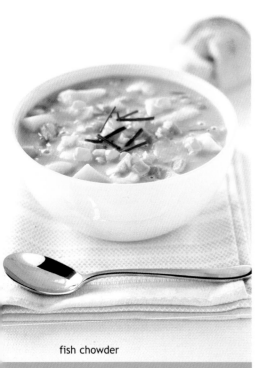

fish chowder

fabulous fish

▶ Fish is an excellent source of high-quality protein, which assists in strengthening and maintaining muscles, and repairing tissue damage. It is also a good source of Omega-3 fatty acids, which are important for good health.

▶ Fresh fish fillets should have a pleasant sea smell — coastal areas are usually the best place to find fresh fish.

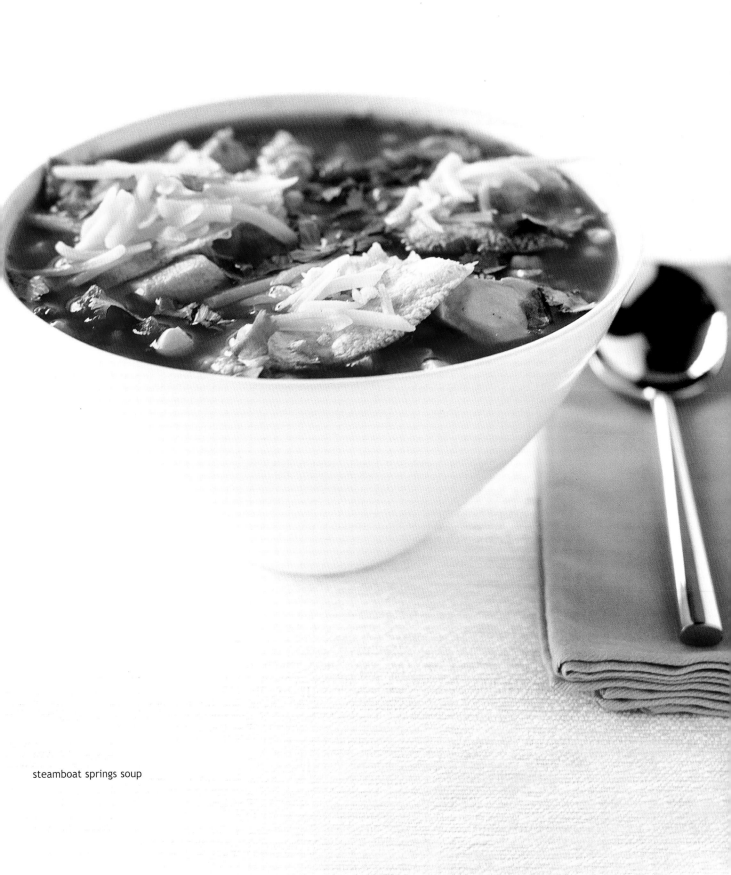

steamboat springs soup

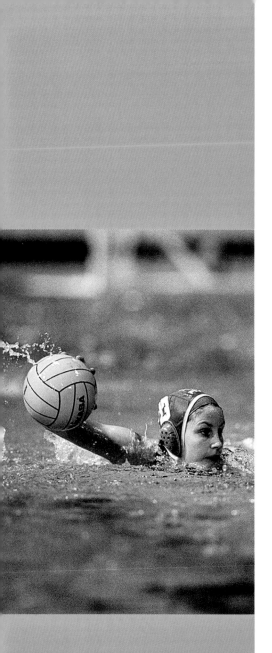

turkey stirfry with couscous Serves 4-6 ✷

3/4-1 cup couscous
300g sweet potato, peeled and cubed
olive or canola oil spray
1 onion, sliced
500g turkey breast or cutlets, sliced

250g green beans, sliced into
  3cm pieces
1 cup halved yellow squash
250g jar cranberry sauce
100g frozen cranberries (optional)

Cover couscous with 2 cups boiling water and set aside. Heat sweet potato in microwave on HIGH for 2-3 minutes or until soft, set aside. Spray a non-stick frypan or wok with oil and cook onion over medium heat for 5 minutes or until golden. Add turkey and cook until browned. Transfer to a bowl. Add beans to pan/wok and stirfry for 1 minute. Add squash, cranberry sauce, sweet potato, onion and turkey. Stir until cranberry sauce is mixed through, then cook for a further 2 minutes. Add cranberries, if desired, and stir through. Fluff couscous with a fork and serve with stirfry.

Analysis	High Fuel	Low Fuel
	4	6
energy (kj)	2673	1588
• protein (g)	40	25
• fat (g)	8	5
• CHO (g)	99	56
• vitamin C		

mustard burgers with coleslaw Makes 8 ✷

olive or canola oil spray
1 onion, finely diced
2 tsp minced garlic
1 tsp minced chilli
600g premium beef mince
1 tbs wholegrain mustard
2 tbs tomato paste
2 tbs finely chopped gherkins
2 tbs chopped fresh chives
freshly ground black pepper
8 hamburger buns

mustard and tomato sauce, to serve

coleslaw:
200g white cabbage, chopped
200g red cabbage, chopped
1 large carrot, grated
2 sticks celery, finely chopped
1 small red capsicum, deseeded
  and finely chopped
1/2 cup low-fat coleslaw dressing
2 tbs chopped fresh chives

To make coleslaw, combine all ingredients in a large bowl. Refrigerate until serving. Spray a non-stick frypan with oil and cook onion, garlic and chilli over medium heat for 5 minutes or until onion is soft. Combine onion mixture with mince, mustard, tomato paste, gherkins and chives, and season with pepper. Shape mixture into 8 patties and refrigerate for 15-30 minutes. Cook patties in a non-stick frypan over medium heat for 8 minutes, then turn and cook for 5 minutes more or until cooked through. Serve the patties with buns, mustard, tomato sauce and coleslaw.

Analysis	High Fuel	Low Fuel
	2 burgers	1 burger
energy (kj)	3208	1604
• protein (g)	48	24
• fat (g)	20	10
• CHO (g)	90	45
• iron, vitamin C		

amy hetzel —
water polo player

"When we travel to the United States, we always stay in hotels, which means we rely on eating out for our meals. The biggest problem we face is having access to suitable snack choices between meals. I always pack my own supply of favourite snack choices, including rice cakes, tinned fruit, a liquid meal supplement and dried fruit-and-nut mix."

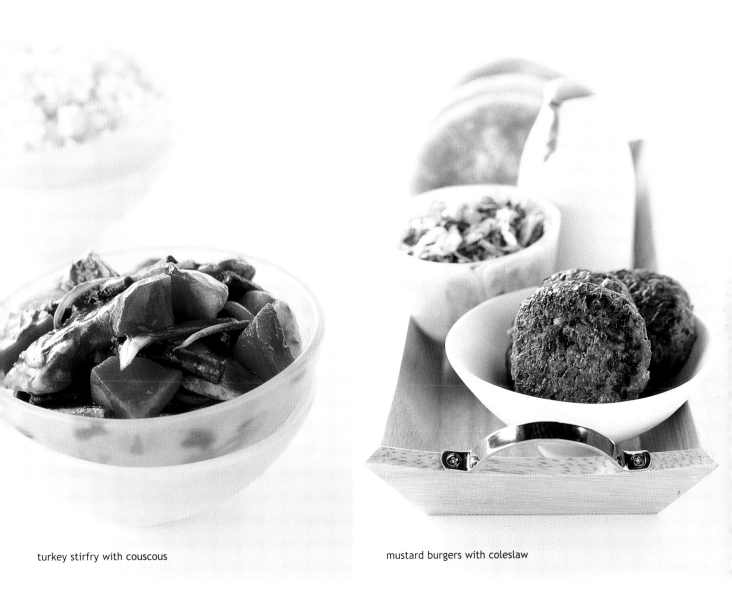

turkey stirfry with couscous

mustard burgers with coleslaw

"A little bit of creativity and flexibility is necessary when trying to cook delicious meals away from home. Test my skills for yourself by trying Barney's Blended Juice." (See recipe, page 32.)

— paul 'barney' matthews, triathlete

mini new york cheesecakes Makes 8

6 wheatmeal biscuits, crumbled
200g low-fat ricotta cheese
125g light cream cheese, softened
1/2 cup NESTLÉ Sweetened
   Condensed Skim Milk

1/3 cup caster sugar
3 eggwhites
200g mixed fresh blueberries
   and raspberries

Analysis	8 serves
energy (kj)	812
protein (g)	8
fat (g)	6
CHO (g)	28
calcium	

Preheat oven to 180°C (350°F). Line eight holes in a 12-hole muffin pan with paper muffin cases. Place crumbled biscuits in the base of each case. Beat together cheeses, condensed milk, sugar and eggwhites. Spoon into cases and bake for 25 minutes or until set. Allow to cool. Serve topped with berries.

date cookies Makes 38

50g butter or margarine, softened
grated rind of 1 orange
3/4 cup caster sugar
1 egg
1 cup plain flour

1/2 tsp bicarbonate of soda
2/3 cup desiccated coconut
100g chopped pitted dates
1/2 cup low-fat sour cream

Preheat oven to 180°C (350°F). Line 4 baking trays with non-stick paper. Beat butter or margarine, orange rind and sugar until well combined. Add egg and beat until combined. Stir in flour, bicarbonate of soda and coconut. Mix in dates, breaking up any clumps. Add sour cream and mix until just combined. Place rounded teaspoons of mixture on trays about 2-3cm apart. Bake 2 trays of cookies at a time, for 15-20 minutes or until lightly browned. Cool for 5 minutes on tray, then transfer to a rack.

Analysis	Per biscuit
energy (kj)	280
protein (g)	1
fat (g)	3
CHO (g)	10

Option: Combine 1/2 cup icing sugar and 2 teaspoons orange juice. Drizzle over cooled biscuits.

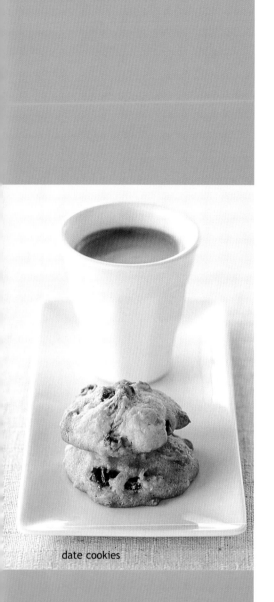

date cookies

make it a date

▶ Dates have been cultivated for at least 5,000 years. They are a great snack food and make a delicious sweet addition to cakes, biscuits, slices and loaves.

▶ Although packaged dates are tougher and not as sweet as fresh dates, they tend to be better for cooking. If you do use fresh dates, avoid overcooking so they don't become mushy in the biscuit.

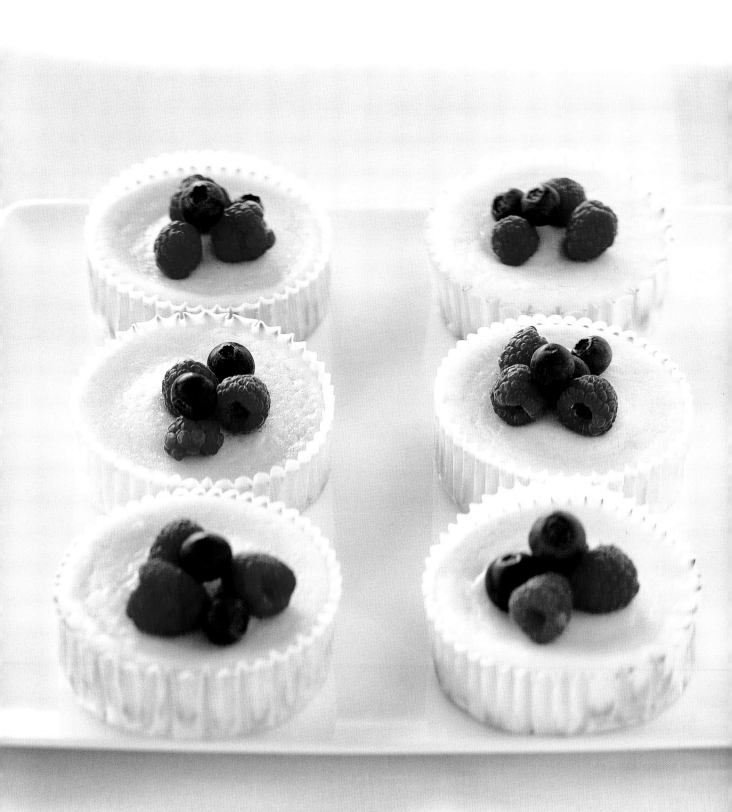

mini new york cheesecakes

central america

Throughout Central America, meat, seafood and vegetables are prepared in myriad ways, with beans, onions and peppers used liberally and rice served as a staple. One of the region's most versatile inventions is tortillas — use them as a savoury base or sweeten them up by adding sugar and spices, and serving them with fruit.

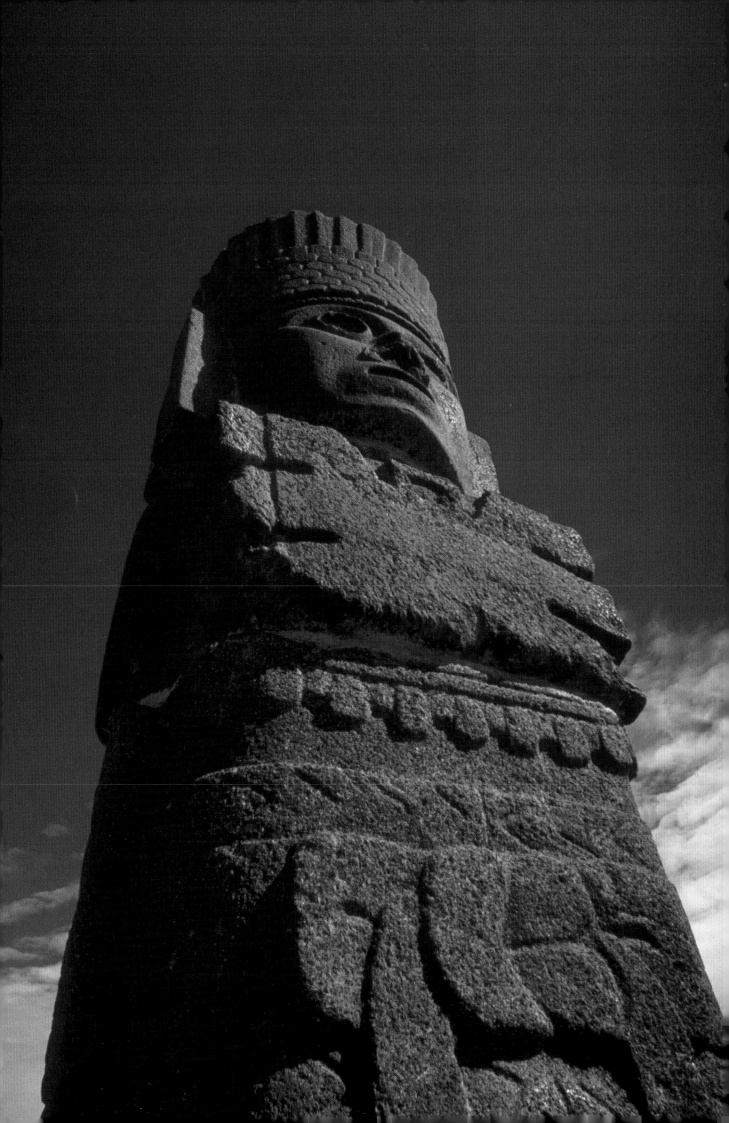

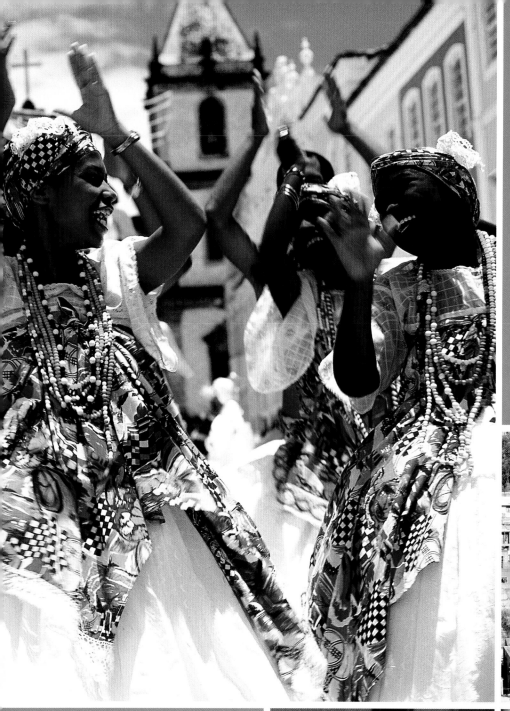

food availability

City dwellers in this region have access to a variety of international and traditional foods. Those athletes who need to be conservative with their food choices will find many western-style establishments that can cater for them. Street vendors sell an enticing array of traditional foods but are probably best avoided when training and competing are a priority. Food availability decreases in more isolated areas so taking some supplies may help you avoid local delicacies, such as chapulines (grasshoppers). Supermarkets and markets provide basic supplies for self-catering, however some foods, such as quality breakfast cereals, cereal bars and sports foods, will be hard to source.

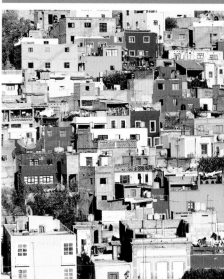

about the culture

The cuisine of Central America is colourful, deeply flavoured and often spicy. Rice, maize, beans, chicken, eggs, fish and tropical fruit feature widely. Flavoursome soups, stews and casseroles are popular, as are small portions of meat and vegetables wrapped in either tortillas (e.g. enchiladas), pastry (empanadas) or corn husks (tamales). In general, the further north you travel the spicier the food becomes, with Mexico providing the fieriest menus. Food tends to become more meat-based as you head towards South America, and potatoes take prominence over rice and maize. Breakfast in this region often consists of sweet, deep-fried pastry or egg dishes served with thick coffee, chocolate or sweetened milk. Lunch is the main meal of the day and is typically followed by a siesta. Dinner is often eaten quite late (after 9pm).

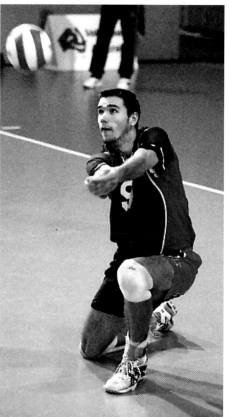

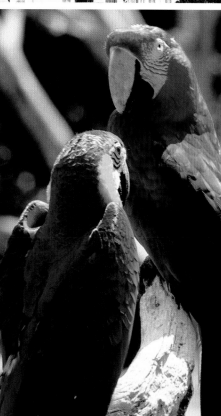

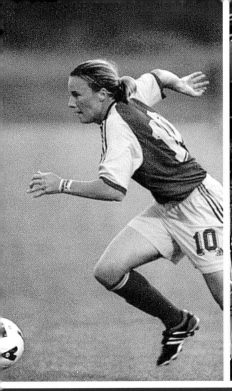

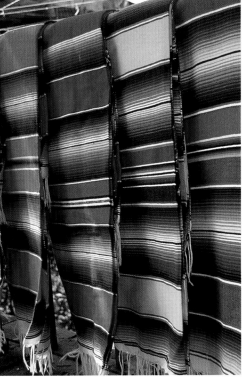

useful tips

- Care needs to be taken with food hygiene. Many AIS athletes have fallen ill when travelling within this area
- It is important to drink extra fluid when visiting countries with a high altitude
- Appetite can decrease when altitude increases. Try to have small, regular snacks if you are unable to eat your regular-sized meals
- Mexican foods are often much hotter than those available in western-style Mexican restaurants. Even avid chilli lovers should be conservative. Enchiladas, quesadillas, tostadas or beans and rice are likely to be safer options, however you will need to check the fillings
- If you find yourself 'enjoying' a little too much chilli, try having some milk or yogurt. The casein (protein) is thought to reduce the discomfort. Other liquids, such as water, only provide a temporary fix.

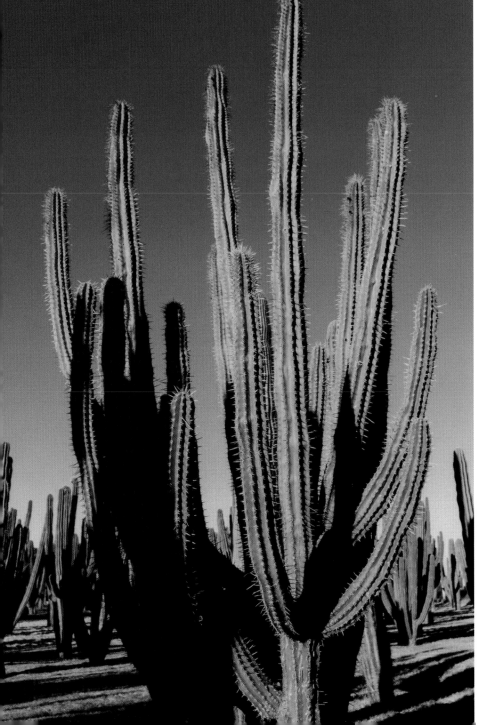

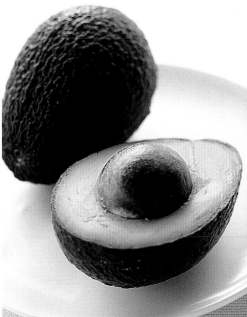

main nutrient sources

carbohydrate
Rice, beans, corn, tortillas, potato, fruit and juice are good options

protein
Beans, chicken, eggs, beef and fish (from safe suppliers only)

fat
Beware of mixed-meat grills, deep-fried pastries and high-fat desserts.

central america

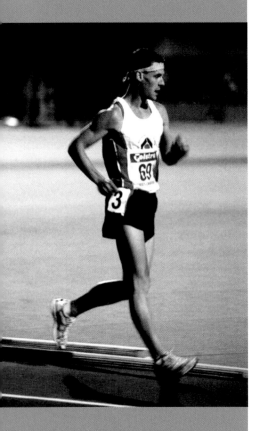

nathan deakes — walker

"I suggest staying away from street stalls in Mexico, but if you really want to try a 'typical' Mexican meal, head for a comedor. They offer Mexico's cheapest sit-down meals. Choose wisely — look for one that is busy and prepares food in front of you. It's best to go at lunchtime when ingredients are at their freshest."

calamari salad   Serves 4-6

1-1½ cups couscous
½ cup red wine vinegar
2 tsp minced garlic
2 tbs olive oil
500g calamari tubes, cleaned and
　cut into rings
1 cup chopped celery

1 small cucumber, chopped
1 each small red, green and yellow
　capsicum, deseeded and cut into
　long, thin strips
3 green shallots, chopped
2 tbs chopped fresh flat-leaf parsley
1 finely chopped fresh jalapeño chilli

Cover couscous with 3 cups boiling water and allow to stand. Mix vinegar, garlic and oil in a small bowl. Bring 1 cup water to a low boil in a frypan. Stir in squid and cook for 2 minutes or until opaque and tender. Drain and cool. Mix celery, cucumber, capsicums, green shallots, parsley and chilli in a large bowl. Gently toss with squid and dressing. Refrigerate until serving. Fluff couscous with a fork and serve with squid.

Analysis	High Fuel	Low Fuel
	4	6
energy (kj)	2690	1406
● protein (g)	37	22
● fat (g)	12	8
● CHO (g)	93	43
● iron, vitamin C		

beef fajitas   Serves 4-6

1 cup rice (omit for Low Fuel)
1 tsp minced garlic
3 tbs barbecue sauce
2 tbs MAGGI Chilli Sauce
1 tsp ground cumin
1 tsp ground coriander
500g beef, cut into strips
250g cherry tomatoes, quartered
400g can corn kernels,
　rinsed and drained
1 Lebanese cucumber, diced

2 tbs lemon juice
olive or canola oil spray
1 red onion, sliced
1 red capsicum, deseeded and sliced
200g button mushrooms, sliced
1 tbs chopped bottled jalapeño chillies
2 tbs chopped fresh coriander
12 flour tortillas
12 lettuce leaves
taco sauce, to serve

Cook rice according to packet instructions (omit for Low Fuel). Combine garlic, sauces, spices and beef in a plastic bag. Massage to evenly coat meat. Refrigerate for 15-30 minutes to marinate. Meanwhile, to make a salsa, combine tomatoes, corn, cucumber and lemon juice in a small bowl. Spray a non-stick frypan with oil and cook onion, capsicum and mushrooms over medium-high heat until soft. Add meat and cook until browned. Stir through chillies and coriander. Heat tortillas in microwave on HIGH for 30-60 seconds or until warm and flexible. To assemble fajitas, line tortillas with lettuce, top with meat mixture, salsa and taco sauce and roll up. Serve with rice.

Analysis	High Fuel	Low Fuel
	4	6
energy (kj)	3285	1686
● protein (g)	44	27
● fat (g)	13	8
● CHO (g)	116	50
● calcium, iron, vitamin C		

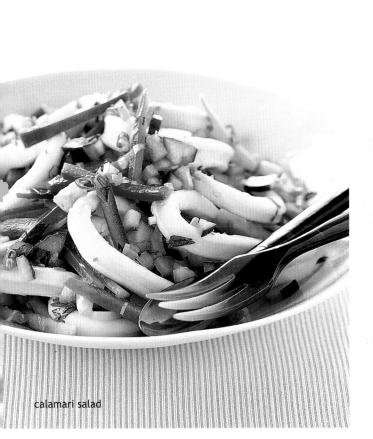

calamari salad

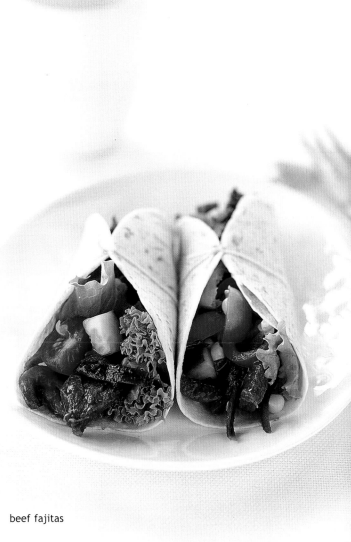

beef fajitas

"We travel to some out-of-the-way places, where food availability is challenging. Cooking for ourselves is the best option — except when your team-mates create cabbage cooked in gherkin juice with gherkins on top!"

— robin bell, canoe slalom

mexican chicken baskets Serves 4-6 ❄

12 enchilada tortillas
olive or canola oil spray
500g chicken mince
1 red capsicum, deseeded and
   finely chopped
440g can kidney beans,
   rinsed and drained
200g Mexican salsa

1 punnet grape or cherry tomatoes,
   quartered
minced chilli (optional)
freshly ground black pepper
1 packet gourmet salad lettuce leaves
300g can corn kernels,
   rinsed and drained
grated low-fat cheese, to serve

Preheat oven to 180°C (350°F). Heat tortillas in microwave on HIGH for 30-60 seconds or until warm and flexible. Spray one side of each with oil and arrange, sprayed-side down, in a muffin pan to form little baskets. Keep openings and sides of baskets wide to allow them to hold as much filling as possible. Bake for 7-10 minutes or until golden brown, then leave in tray while cooling to keep their shape. Spray a non-stick frypan with oil and cook mince over high heat for 5 minutes or until browned, using a wooden spoon to break up any lumps. Add capsicum, beans, salsa and tomatoes and heat through. Add chilli, if desired, and pepper, to taste, and simmer for 5-10 minutes or until sauce thickens. Line baskets with lettuce leaves and top with a large spoonful of chicken mixture. Sprinkle with corn and cheese.

Analysis	High Fuel	Low Fuel
	4	6
energy (kj)	3009	2006
protein (g)	53	36
fat (g)	15	10
CHO (g)	79	53
calcium, iron, vitamin C		

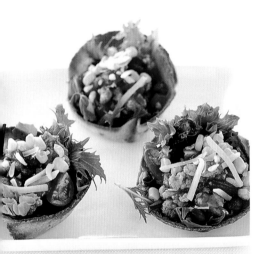

mexican chicken baskets

the best tortilla baskets

▶ The easiest way to ensure that your baskets don't break up is to warm up the tortillas before cooking. You can do this by placing them in the microwave for 30-60 seconds or by wrapping them in foil and placing in the oven or under the grill for 10 minutes.

▶ Cook the Mexican Chicken Baskets until crisp and golden — don't remove them from the oven too early or the baskets won't hold together.

mexican rice Serves 4-6 ❄

olive or canola oil spray
1 small onion, diced
1 tsp minced garlic
1 tsp minced chilli
1¹/2-2 cups long-grain
   white rice
1/2 cup tomato puree

3 cups MAGGI Real Chicken Stock
2 carrots, diced
1/2 cup fresh or frozen peas
420g can four bean mix,
   rinsed and drained
1/2 cup blanched almonds

Analysis	High Fuel	Low Fuel
	4	6
energy (kj)	2669	1527
protein (g)	21	13
fat (g)	13	8
CHO (g)	103	55
iron		

Spray a non-stick saucepan with oil and cook onion, garlic and chilli over medium heat until soft. Add rice and cook, stirring, for 2 minutes. Add tomato puree and cook for a further 2-3 minutes. Add stock and bring to the boil, then add vegetables and beans. Reduce heat to low, cover and simmer for 15 minutes. Stir in almonds and heat through.

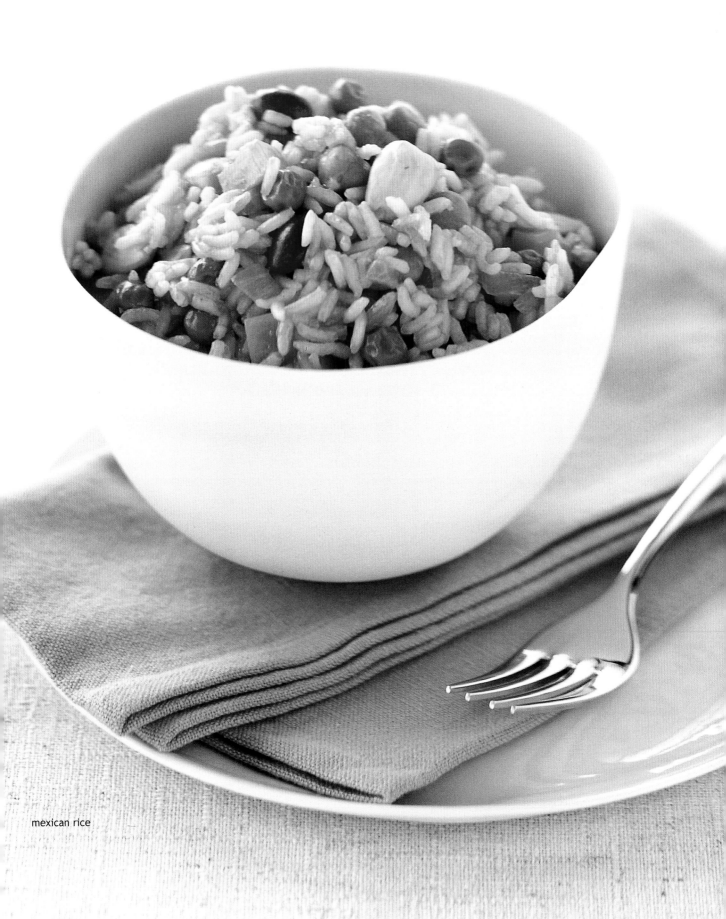

mexican rice

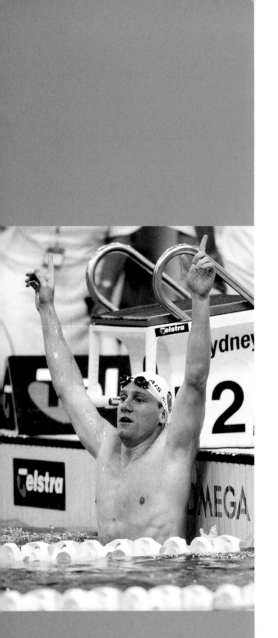

regan harrison —
swimmer

"I have travelled the globe with swimming. I've eaten in some of the best restaurants and sampled the cuisine of numerous countries. On a trip to Mexico, I realised just how good it is to cook your own Mexican at home! We were told to eat in the restaurant in the team hotel and to use bottled water for everything. But even so, many guys on the team got tummy bugs. It's the less glamorous part of travel!"

tortilla lasagne Serves 4-8 ✳

olive or canola oil spray
1 onion, finely chopped
500g extra-lean beef mince
1 packet MAGGI Chilli Con Carne
    Recipe Mix
300g can corn kernels,
    rinsed and drained
435g can refried beans

400g can crushed tomatoes
600g chunky salsa
8 large burrito flour tortillas
450g frozen spinach, defrosted and
    excess water squeezed out
1/2 cup grated reduced-fat cheese
salad leaves, to serve

Preheat oven to 200°C (400°F). Spray a non-stick saucepan with oil and cook onion over medium heat until soft. Add mince and cook until browned. Add chilli con carne mix, corn, refried beans, tomatoes and two-thirds of salsa. Stir, bring to the boil, then reduce heat and simmer for 10 minutes or until sauce thickens. Place a little meat sauce in the base of a 29cm x 23cm lasagne dish. Top with about 4 tortillas, then add alternate layers of meat sauce, spinach and tortillas, finishing with a tortilla layer. Spread remaining salsa over the top. Sprinkle with cheese and bake for 25-30 minutes or until cheese is melted and golden brown. Allow to stand for 10 minutes before slicing. Serve with salad leaves.

Analysis	High Fuel	Low Fuel
	4	8
energy (kj)	3266	1633
protein (g)	53	26
fat (g)	21	11
CHO (g)	85	43
calcium, iron, vitamin C		

chicken & cashew tostadas Serves 4-6

1 1/2 cups spiral pasta
    (omit for Low Fuel)
1 sweet potato, peeled and
    cut into 1.5-2cm cubes
3 tomatoes, diced
2 Lebanese cucumbers, diced
400g can pineapple pieces in natural
    juice, drained and diced
freshly ground black pepper
olive or canola oil spray
500g chicken tenderloins or skinless
    chicken breast fillets, sliced

1 onion, finely chopped
1 red capsicum, deseeded and
    cut into small strips
60g unsalted cashew nuts
juice of 1 lemon
12 enchilada tortillas
1 iceberg lettuce
200g Mexican salsa
200g PETERS FARM Natural
    No Fat Set Yogurt
chopped fresh coriander leaves,
    to serve

Cook pasta according to packet instructions (omit for Low Fuel). Cook sweet potato in microwave for 5 minutes on HIGH or until soft. Combine tomatoes, cucumbers and pineapple in a small bowl to make a salsa. Season with pepper and set aside. Spray a non-stick wok with oil and stirfry chicken in batches over medium-high heat until browned. Set aside. Add onion to wok and cook until soft. Add capsicum, cashews, pasta, chicken and sweet potato, and stirfry until chicken is tender. Season with lemon juice and pepper. Meanwhile, heat tortillas in microwave on HIGH for 30-60 seconds or until warm and flexible. To assemble, place 2 tortillas on a plate, overlapping in centre. Cover with lettuce leaves, then spoonfuls of stirfry mix and homemade salsa. Top with a dollop each of Mexican salsa and yogurt and sprinkle with coriander.

Analysis	High Fuel	Low Fuel
	4	6
energy (kj)	3138	1582
protein (g)	47	27
fat (g)	17	11
CHO (g)	93	38
calcium, iron, vitamin C		

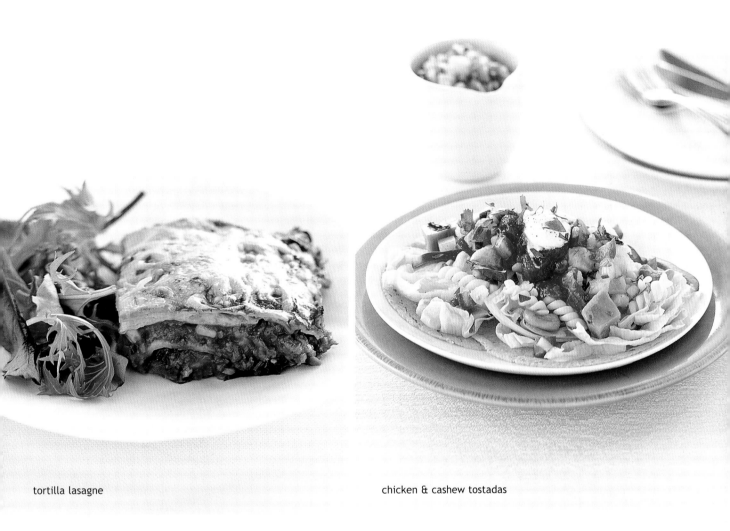

tortilla lasagne

chicken & cashew tostadas

"I've had my meals provided by the AIS dining hall for the past four years. Fortunately, regular cooking classes with our dietitian mean I can also fend for myself if necessary."

— jacqui dunn, gymnast

fruity salsa tortillas Serves 4

4 large burrito flour tortillas
1 eggwhite, lightly beaten
caster sugar, to sprinkle,
   plus 2 tsp extra
ground cinnamon, to sprinkle
250g strawberries, hulled and chopped
2 fresh mangoes, flesh chopped
(or 1 x 400g can chopped mango
   slices if unavailable)
2 kiwifruit, peeled and chopped
pulp of 4 passionfruit (or 170g can
   passionfruit in syrup if unavailable)
4 scoops PETERS Light & Creamy
   Ice-cream

Preheat oven to 180°C (350°F). Heat tortillas in microwave on HIGH for 30-60 seconds or until warm and flexible, then brush one side of each with eggwhite and sprinkle with sugar and cinnamon. Cut in half. Fold each half into a cone shape, sprinkled-side folded inwards. Stand in a muffin pan, wide-side down, and bake in oven for 7-10 minutes or until brown. Leave to cool in pan. Meanwhile, combine strawberries, mangoes, kiwifruit and half the passionfruit pulp in a bowl to make a fruit salsa. Sprinkle with a little cinnamon. Combine remaining passionfruit pulp with a little water and extra 2 teaspoons sugar. (If using passionfruit in syrup, use straight from can – do not add water and sugar.) Spoon salsa into cones and lay on a plate. Pour passionfruit mixture over the top. Serve with ice-cream.

Analysis	4 serves
energy (kj)	1034
protein (g)	8
● fat (g)	2
● CHO (g)	43
● vitamin C	

fruity salsa tortillas

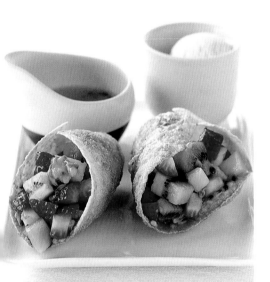

chilli chocolate mousse Serves 6

500ml low-fat custard
400g NESTLÉ All Natural 99% Fat Free
   Vanilla Yogurt
1/2 tsp chilli powder (optional)
1 cup NESQUIK Chocolate Powder
1/2 cup icing sugar
3 tsp powdered gelatine
2 eggwhites
200g mixed fresh berries (optional)
50g grated NESTLÉ Smooth 'n'
   Creamy Milk Chocolate

Whisk custard, yogurt, chilli, NESQUIK and icing sugar in a bowl until combined. Combine gelatine and 3 tablespoons water in a small saucepan and stir over low heat until gelatine dissolves and liquid is clear. Remove from heat and allow to cool slightly. Beat eggwhites in a clean, dry bowl until soft peaks form. Fold eggwhites and gelatine mixture through chocolate mixture. Divide between 6 serving glasses and refrigerate until set. Serve topped with berries, if desired, and chocolate.

Tip: For a plain chocolate mousse, omit chilli powder.

Analysis	6 serves
energy (kj)	1296
● protein (g)	11
● fat (g)	4
● CHO (g)	57
● calcium	

tortilla treats

▶ For a different flavour, you can replace the sugar and cinnamon in the Fruity Salsa Tortillas with nutmeg and mixed spice.

▶ There are various ways to use tortillas. They are deliciously refreshing when filled with fruit but you can also use them as a casing for ice-cream or as an accompaniment to ice-cream sundaes or banana splits.

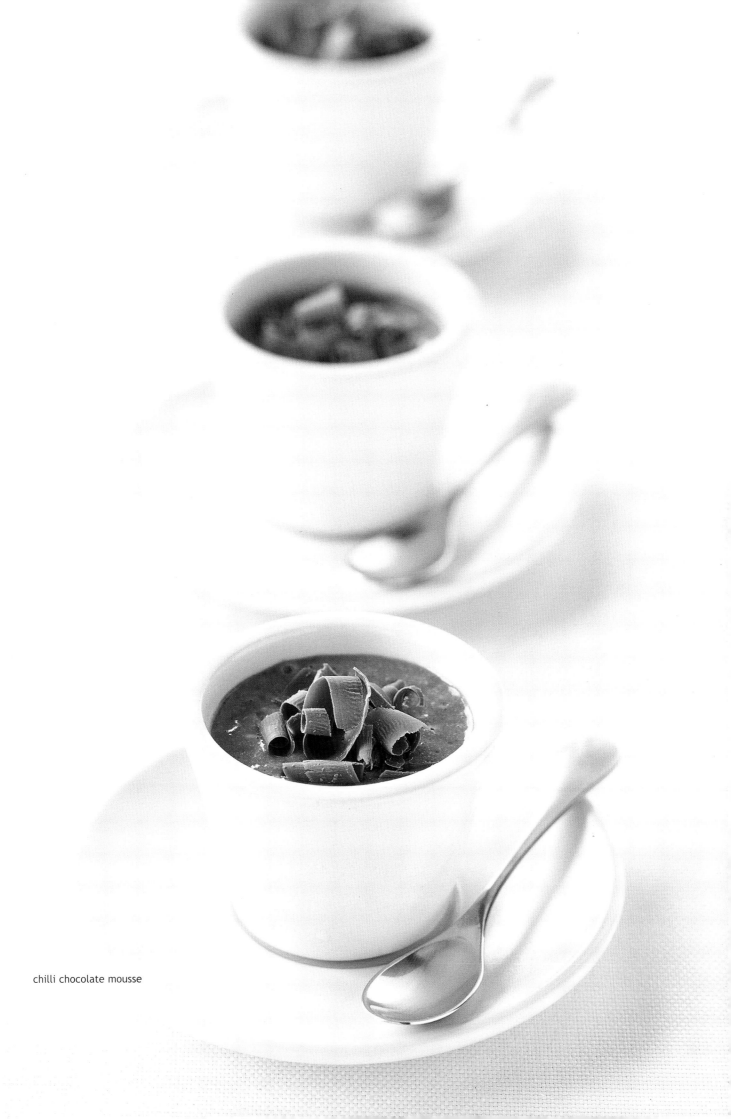

chilli chocolate mousse

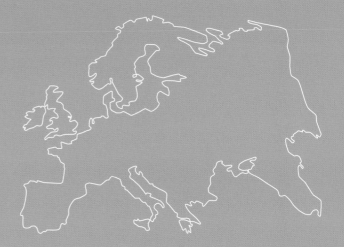

europe

The extraordinary array of cultures that makes up Europe presents visitors with endless culinary options. The idea is to embrace local traditions and sample the dishes each country is most famous for — try pasta in Italy, paella in Spain, moussaka and souvlaki in Greece and a hearty stroganoff or schnitzel in central Europe.

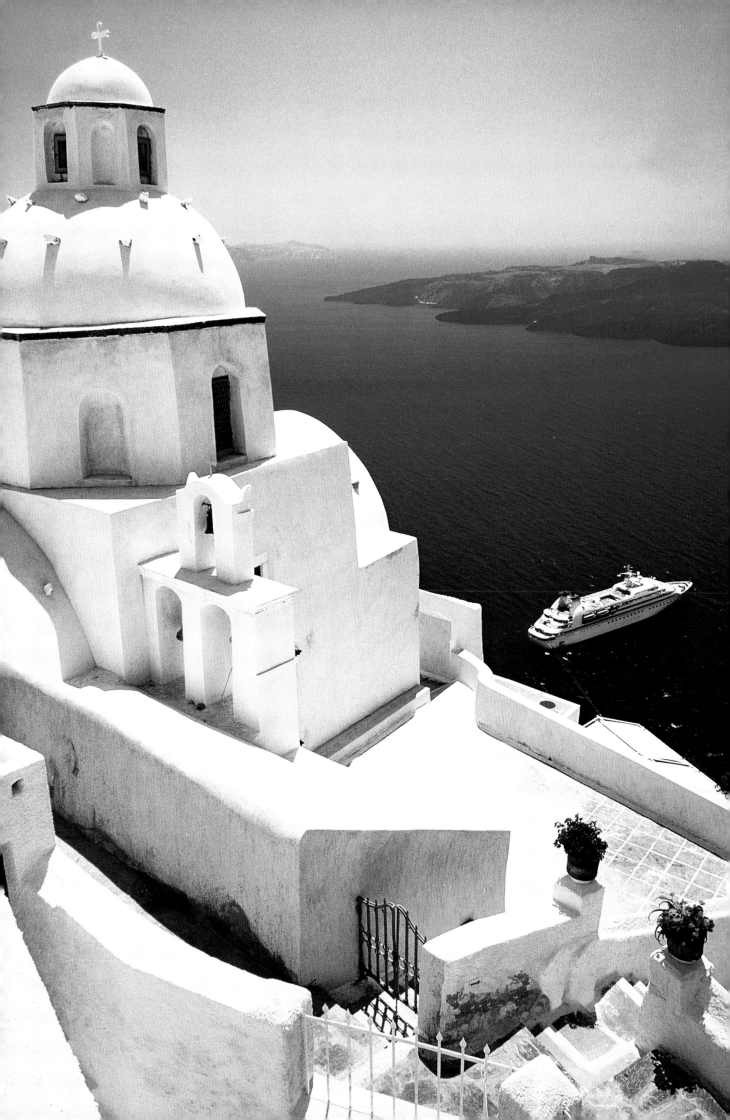

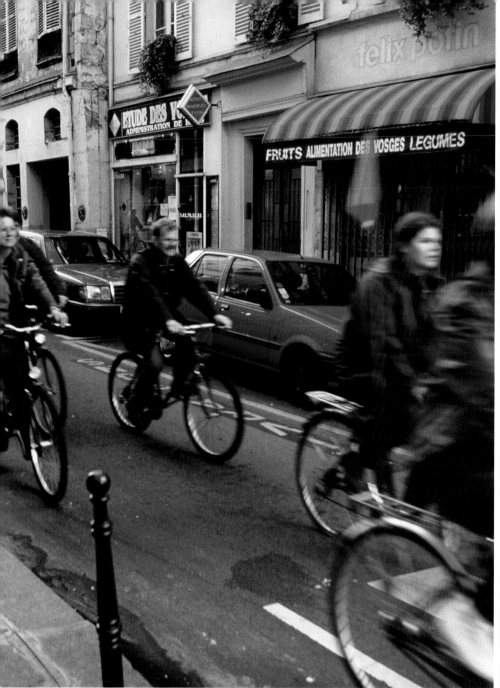

food availability

Restaurant dining tends to be quite formal throughout Europe. Some restaurants will prepare special dishes on request, but it is worth calling in advance if you have special dietary needs (e.g. vegetarian, gluten-free). International cuisine has infiltrated many European countries, particularly in the major cities. Austria, for instance, has many Asian restaurants and pizzerias, while the Netherlands has numerous Indonesian and Turkish restaurants due to the influence of immigration from these countries. Self-catering is relatively easy throughout most of Europe and is certainly more economical than relying on restaurants. Food availability is limited in eastern Europe, particularly for fresh fruit and vegetables. Sports foods are available throughout most of western Europe though brands vary, but they can be hard to find in some parts of eastern Europe.

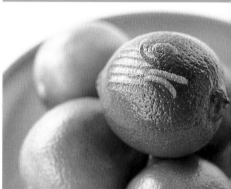

about the culture

Europe offers a diverse variety of cuisines. Western European cuisine usually includes many vegetables and salads, as well as seafood, meat and poultry. Cuisine in eastern Europe and Germany tends to be based on large amounts of meat, and fresh vegetables are harder to come by. Throughout Europe, breakfast tends to differ from the typical Australian athlete breakfast. In some countries, it is a light meal – coffee and tostada (buttered toast) in Spain, or coffee and a pastry in Belgium. In other countries, much larger meals are the norm – wurst (sausage) with cheese and bread in Germany, burek (greasy layered pie with meat and cheese) in Croatia, or a large fry-up in the UK. In many countries, lunch is the main meal of the day and a lighter evening meal is eaten as late as 10 or 11pm.

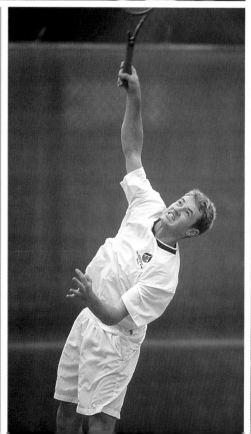

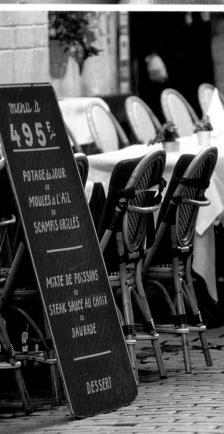

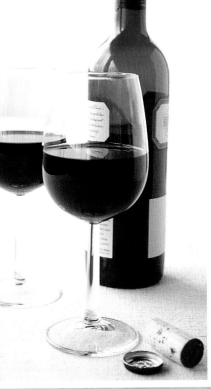

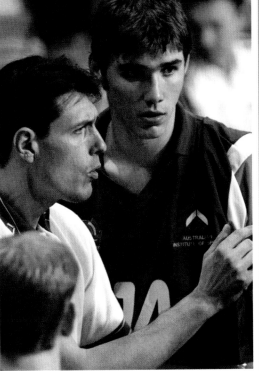

useful tips:

- ▶ When asking for water in restaurants, cafés and shops, you should specify if you want tap water. Most restaurants will provide more expensive bottled mineral water as the standard choice
- ▶ Beware of 'tourist menus'. They are usually more expensive
- ▶ Meal sizes vary considerably throughout Europe. Belgium, Germany and the Netherlands are notorious for providing very large portions.

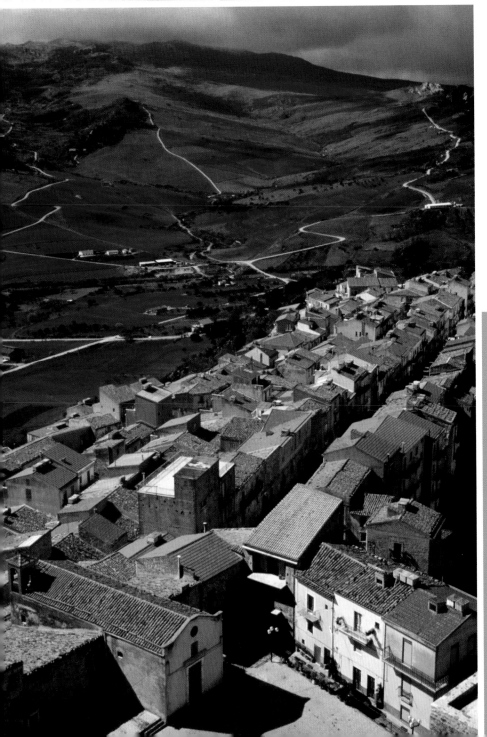

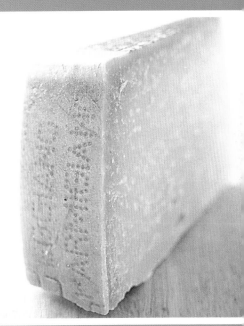

main nutrient sources

carbohydrate
Pasta, rice, potatoes and numerous varieties of bread rolls and bread are available throughout Europe

protein
A wide variety of meats, poultry and seafood are available in most countries. Meals in Spain and Portugal tend to focus on seafood. Cheese and eggs are also abundant in the majority of regions

fat
High-fat cheeses are used widely in many European countries. Swiss meals, in particular, are notorious for containing high-fat cheeses in most recipes. It is useful to ask what ingredients are used in the rich sauces and soups that are so common throughout Europe, as a large proportion of these will be high in fat. Wurst, a staple in the German diet, makes the fat content of many German dishes extra high.

europe

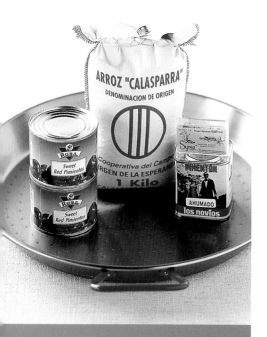

saffron chicken paella Serves 4-6 ✳

olive or canola oil spray
500g chicken breast fillets, cubed
2 tsp minced garlic
1 red onion, sliced
1 each red and green capsicum,
   deseeded and chopped
1 1/3-2 cups short-grain rice
3 ripe tomatoes, chopped

200g green beans, chopped
2 tsp sweet paprika
3-4 cups MAGGI Real Chicken Stock
1/2 tsp saffron threads
400g can chickpeas,
   rinsed and drained
1 cup frozen peas

Spray a large non-stick frypan or paella pan with oil and cook chicken over medium heat until browned. Add garlic, onion and capsicums and cook for 3 minutes or until softened. Add rice, tomatoes, beans and paprika and cook for 2 minutes. Add stock and saffron, bring to the boil, then reduce heat to low and simmer, without stirring, for 15 minutes. Shake pan a couple of times during cooking to stop rice from sticking. Stir in chickpeas and peas and cook for 3 minutes or until heated through.

Analysis	High Fuel	Low Fuel
	4	6
energy (kj)	3111	1702
protein (g)	48	30
fat (g)	12	7
CHO (g)	105	51
iron, vitamin C		

sherwood pie Serves 4-6 ✳

1/2 cup textured vegetable protein
   (TVP) mince
800g can chopped tomatoes
150g tomato paste
2 carrots, peeled and diced
2 zucchini, diced
8 button mushrooms, diced
1 onion, diced
1 tsp minced garlic
1 tbs soy sauce
2 tsp MAGGI Sweet Chilli Sauce

2 tbs tomato sauce
1 tsp mixed dried herbs
freshly ground black pepper
4 large potatoes, peeled and boiled
150ml CARNATION Light & Creamy
   Evaporated Milk
2 tbs canola margarine
canola or olive oil spray
1/2 cup grated low-fat cheese
4 large or 6 small bread rolls
tossed salad, to serve (optional)

Preheat oven to 180°C (350°F). Place TVP mince, tomatoes, tomato paste, carrots, zucchini, mushrooms and onion in a large bowl and mix well. Combine garlic, sauces and herbs and add to vegetable mixture. Season with pepper. Set aside for 10-15 minutes or until TVP mince absorbs some liquid. Meanwhile, mash potatoes and add milk and margarine. Continue mashing until the mixture is smooth. Spray a lasagne dish with oil to lightly grease. Place vegetable mixture in lasagne dish, spread the potato mixture over the top and sprinkle with cheese. Bake for 50-60 minutes or until cheese is golden. Sprinkle with pepper and serve with bread rolls and a tossed salad, if desired.

Tip: TVP mince may be replaced with 500g beef mince.

Analysis	High Fuel	Low Fuel
	4	6
energy (kj)	2588	1489
protein (g)	26	16
fat (g)	15	9
CHO (g)	87	48
calcium, iron, vitamin C		

perfect paella

▶ Paella should not be stirred so you get a nice crunchy base. A good paella pan, available at Spanish delis, is worth the investment.

▶ You can use a short to medium-grain rice, but for best results use Spanish paella rice.

▶ If your pan is too big for your cooking surface, place it on top of the barbecue.

▶ For variety, swap the chicken for seafood.

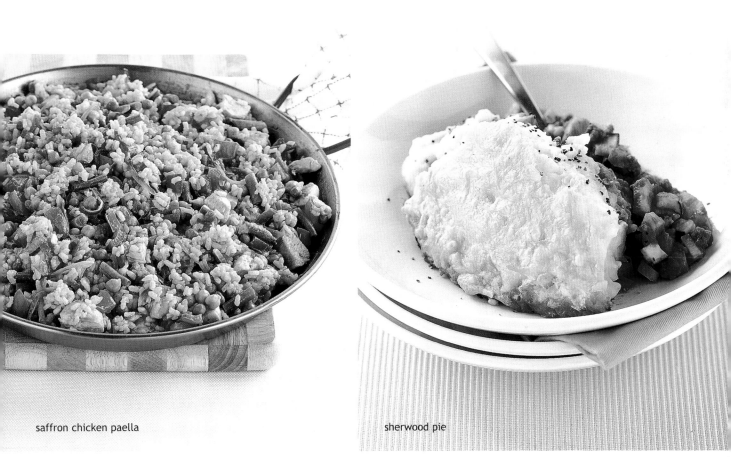

saffron chicken paella

sherwood pie

"Poor organisation before a world track meet in Moscow meant we had to trek 6km in the snow to find food — not the best preparation for a major competition!"
— AIS track cyclists

pork casserole with herb dumplings Serves 4-6 ✳

olive or canola oil spray
500g pork fillet, cubed
200g baby onions, peeled
1 carrot, peeled and thickly sliced
300g pumpkin, peeled, deseeded
  and cubed
1 cup white wine
2 cups MAGGI Real Chicken Stock
2 bay leaves
2 sprigs fresh rosemary
1 red capsicum, deseeded
  and chopped

2 zucchini, sliced
1 tbs cornflour
4-6 corncobs, steamed
4 large bread rolls (omit for Low Fuel)

dumplings:
1 cup self-raising flour,
  plus extra to dust
20g reduced-fat canola margarine
2 tbs chopped fresh herbs (such as
  rosemary, chives, parsley)
1/3 cup skim milk

Spray a large heavy-based saucepan or casserole dish with oil. Add pork and cook over high heat for 3-5 minutes or until browned. Add onions and cook for 5 minutes, until browned. Add carrot, pumpkin, wine, stock, bay leaves and rosemary and bring to the boil. Reduce heat to low and simmer, covered, for 30 minutes. Add capsicum and zucchini and cook for a further 15 minutes. Blend cornflour with 1 tablespoon water and stir into casserole. Cook, stirring, until casserole boils and thickens. Meanwhile, to make dumplings, sift flour into a bowl, then rub in margarine until mixture resembles fine breadcrumbs. Stir in herbs and milk until mixture comes together to form a soft dough. Turn dough out onto a lightly floured surface and gently knead for 1 minute. Divide dough into 8 portions and shape into balls. Place dumplings on top of casserole, then cover and cook over medium heat for 15 minutes or until a skewer inserted into the centre of a dumpling comes out clean. Serve immediately with corncobs and bread rolls. (Omit bread rolls for Low Fuel.)

Analysis	High Fuel	Low Fuel
	4	6
energy (kj)	3025	1524
protein (g)	47	28
fat (g)	12	6
CHO (g)	90	40
iron, vitamin C		

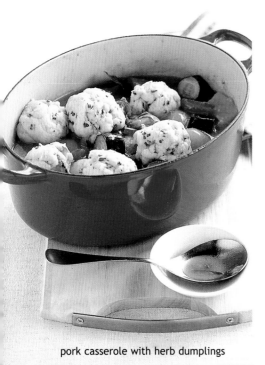

pork casserole with herb dumplings

dumplings to die for

▶ The trick here is to use an enamelled casserole dish made from cast iron — this will prevent the dumplings from sticking to the bottom of the dish and the flavour from being tainted.

▶ Dumplings will only break up when the dough isn't solid. If your dough isn't coming together easily, add a small quantity of liquid.

chicken schnitzel burgers Serves 4 ✳

4 (150g each) single chicken
  breast fillets
1/4 cup plain flour
salt and freshly ground black pepper
2 eggs, lightly beaten
1 tbs skim milk
1 cup dried breadcrumbs

2 tbs chopped fresh flat-leaf parsley
1/4 cup fat-free mayonnaise
200g lettuce mix
2 tomatoes, sliced
1 cucumber, sliced
4 bread rolls (omit for Low Fuel)

Preheat oven to 200°C (400°F). Beat or roll each chicken breast between 2 sheets of plastic wrap until about 1cm thick. Place flour, salt and pepper in a plastic bag and shake until combined. Whisk eggs and milk together in a bowl. Place breadcrumbs and parsley in a separate plastic bag and shake until combined. Place chicken in bag with flour, shake to coat, then shake off excess. Dip chicken in egg mixture, then toss in breadcrumb mixture. Place schnitzels on a baking tray in the freezer for 5 minutes, then bake for 20 minutes or until golden. Assemble burgers with schnitzels, mayonnaise, salad ingredients and bread roll. (For Low Fuel, serve schnitzels with salad only.)

Analysis	High Fuel with bread	Low Fuel no bread
energy (kj)	2853	1959
protein (g)	50	43
fat (g)	19	16
CHO (g)	74	35
iron		

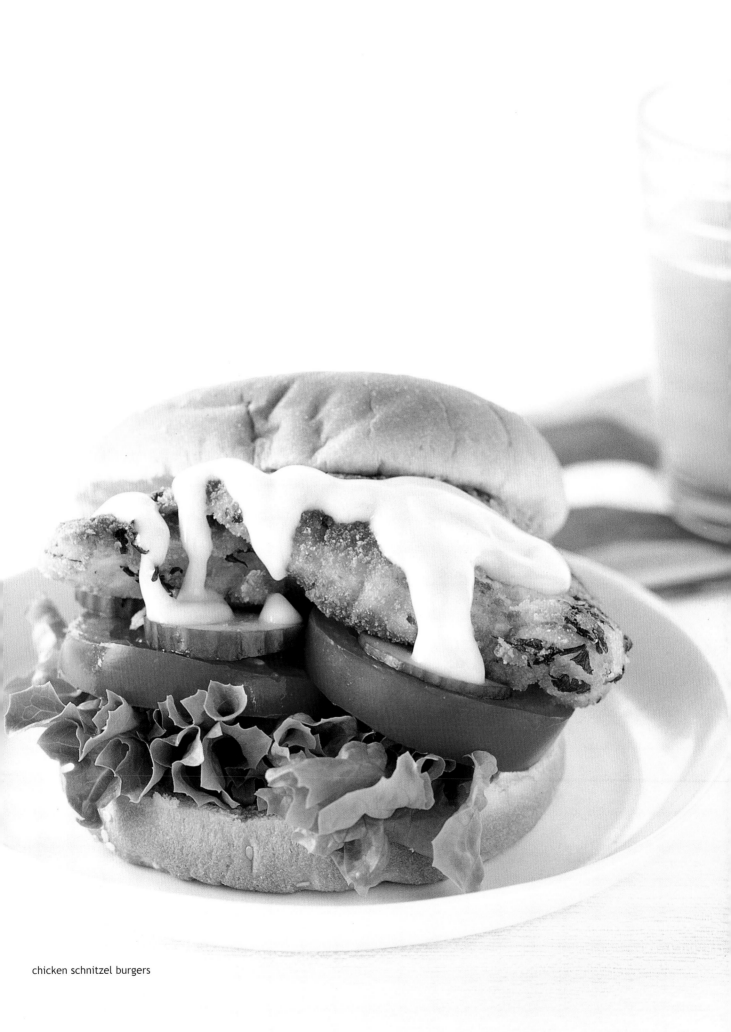

chicken schnitzel burgers

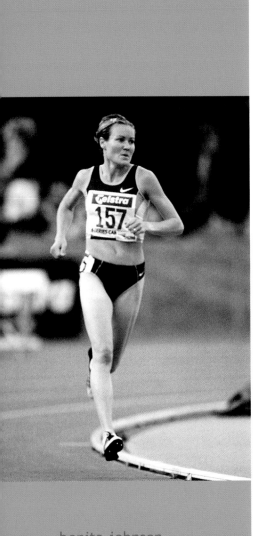

benita johnson – runner

"I spend seven months in the UK each year so I must be aware of what I'm eating. Watch out for the fatty sauces and mayonnaise on pastas and sandwiches. They love their sauces! My advice would be to take over a book from home filled with your favourite recipes – you will not only retain a great diet but save money, too!"

beef stroganoff Serves 4-6 ✳

375-500g fettuccine
400g rump steak
olive or canola oil spray
50g lean bacon, chopped
1 onion, chopped
1 small carrot, peeled and finely sliced
1 stick celery, finely sliced
2 tsp minced garlic
200g button mushrooms, halved
1 tbs plain flour

375ml can CARNATION Light
  & Creamy Evaporated Milk
2 tsp French mustard
1 tsp soy sauce
1/4 cup tomato paste
freshly ground black pepper
fresh flat-leaf parsley leaves,
  to garnish
green salad, to serve

Cook pasta according to packet instructions. Meanwhile, cook steak in a large non-stick frypan over medium-high heat for 3-5 minutes each side or until cooked to your liking. Remove from heat and allow to rest. Reduce heat to medium, spray frypan with oil and cook bacon, onion, carrot, celery, garlic and mushrooms until onion is soft. Add flour and cook, stirring, for 1 minute. Gradually add evaporated milk, then mustard, soy sauce and tomato paste. Bring to the boil, then reduce heat to low and simmer, stirring, until thick. Slice steak into strips, add to pan and heat through. To serve, ladle beef mixture over pasta, sprinkle with pepper and garnish with parsley. Serve with a green salad.

Analysis	High Fuel	Low Fuel
	4	6
energy (kj)	2954	1674
● protein (g)	50	31
● fat (g)	8	5
● CHO (g)	103	55
● calcium, iron		

chocolate raspberry roly poly Serves 6-8

2 cups self-raising flour,
  plus extra to dust
4 tbs NESTLÉ baking cocoa
2/3 cup caster sugar, plus 1/2 cup extra
1 egg, beaten

100-125ml skim milk
raspberry jam, to spread
1 punnet fresh raspberries (or 250g
  frozen raspberries, thawed)
300ml low-fat custard

Preheat oven to 180°C (350°F). Sift flour and 2 tablespoons of the cocoa into a bowl, add 2/3 cup of caster sugar and stir. Make a well in the centre and add egg, stirring, then gradually add milk, stirring, until mixture forms a smooth dough. Turn onto a sheet of baking paper, cover with another sheet of baking paper and roll out to a thin rectangle. The rectangle should be 35-40cm long and just a little shorter in width. Spread jam over the top of dough. Drain berries if necessary and arrange over jam (squash into the jam a little), leaving a 5cm strip down one of the long sides uncovered. Starting from the long edge that is covered with berries, roll up to form a Swiss roll. Transfer to a rectangular cake pan. Combine remaining 2 tablespoons of cocoa and extra 1/2 cup of caster sugar with 11/4 cups boiling water; pour over roll. Bake for 35-40 minutes or until a skewer inserted into the centre comes out clean. Serve with custard.

Analysis	High Fuel	Low Fuel
	6	8
energy (kj)	1783	1337
protein (g)	10	7
● fat (g)	3	2
● CHO (g)	89	67

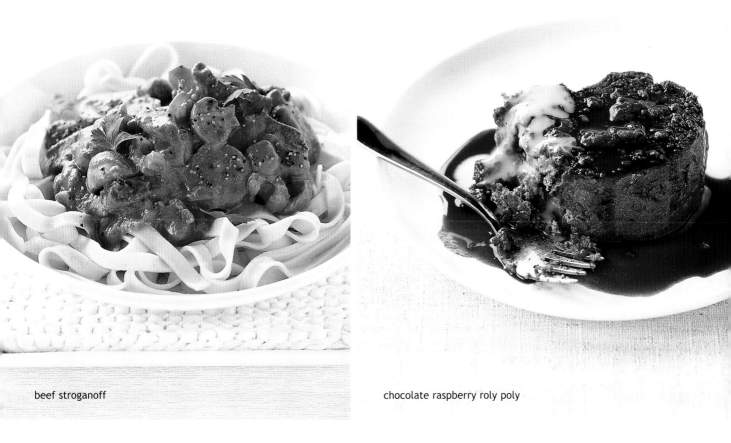

beef stroganoff

chocolate raspberry roly poly

"Last time we competed at Junior Wimbledon our meals were provided at a university residence — meatballs (without pasta), meat loaf and more meat loaf! We ended up having to fend for ourselves in local restaurants."

— chris guccione and adam feeney, tennis players

bircher muesli Serves 4-6

2 cups rolled oats
1/2 cup chopped dried apricots
1 cup orange juice
1 1/2 cups skim milk
1 cup NESTLÉ All Natural 99% Fat Free
  Vanilla Yogurt plus extra, to serve

1/3 cup chopped nuts (such as
  hazelnuts and sliced almonds)
1 apple, grated
honey, to taste
chopped banana or strawberries,
  to serve

Analysis	High Fuel	Low Fuel
	4	6
energy (kj)	1631	1087
protein (g)	15	10
fat (g)	11	7
CHO (g)	55	37
calcium, vitamin C		

Combine oats, apricots, orange juice, milk, yogurt, nuts and apple, cover and refrigerate overnight. Before serving, add honey, to taste. Serve with banana or strawberries and extra yogurt.

lemon self-saucing pudding Serves 4-6

1 cup self-raising flour
3/4 cup caster sugar
1 egg
40g butter, melted
1/2 cup skim milk
grated rind and juice of 2 lemons

1 tbs cornflour
1 tbs custard powder
icing sugar, to serve
PETERS Light & Creamy Ice-cream
  or NESTLÉ All Natural 99% Fat Free
  Vanilla Yogurt, to serve (optional)

Preheat oven to 180°C (350°F). Combine flour and 1/4 cup of the caster sugar in a bowl. Add egg, butter, milk and lemon rind and beat to combine. Pour into a 6-cup capacity ovenproof dish. Combine cornflour, custard powder and the remaining 1/2 cup of caster sugar and sprinkle over top of pudding. Combine lemon juice with 1 1/2 cups boiling water and pour over pudding. Bake pudding for 30-40 minutes or until puffed and golden. Dust with sifted icing sugar and serve with ice-cream or yogurt, if desired.

Analysis	High Fuel	Low Fuel
	4	6
energy (kj)	1649	1099
protein (g)	6	4
fat (g)	10	6
CHO (g)	71	47

Tips: Serve immediately – if you allow the pudding to stand, the sauce will be absorbed back in to the cake. You can substitute the lemon with orange or lime, or try a combination of all three citrus fruits.

bircher muesli

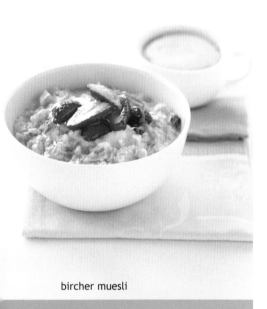

more-ish muesli

▶ Doctor Maximilian Bircher-Benner created this famous dish in the late 1800s at his diet clinic in Switzerland. In 1924 it was named Bircher muesli and became a Swiss national tradition.

▶ Bircher muesli is not only delicious – it is also highly nutritious and easy to make.

▶ You can replace the orange juice with apple juice or reduced-fat milk, if you prefer.

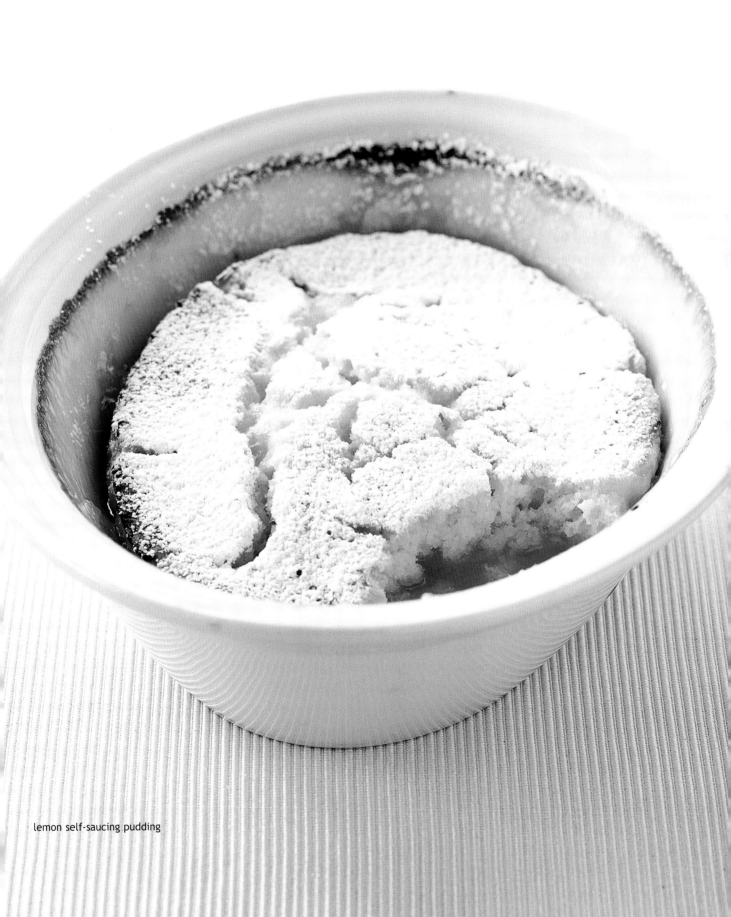

lemon self-saucing pudding

greece

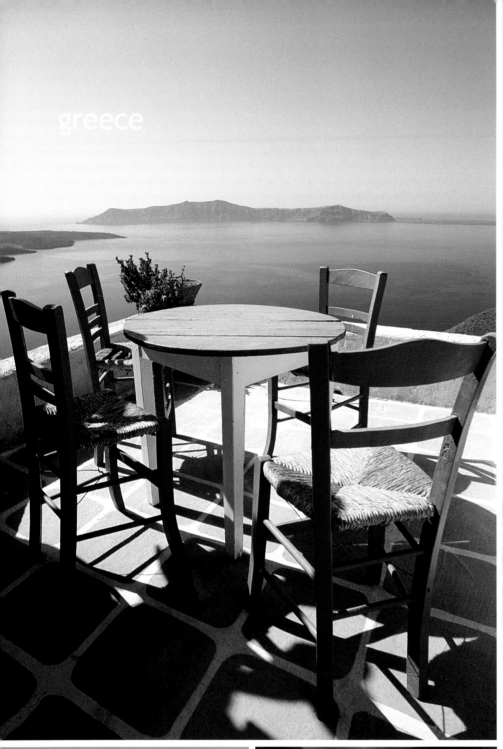

food availability

A variety of eateries, including major franchises, local international restaurants, traditional tavernas and cafés are available throughout Greece. It is common to order 3-4 entrée dishes or mezze when eating out. Traditional mezze include dips, small spicy sausages (loukánika), meatballs (keftédes), dolmades (stuffed vine leaves) and seafood (deep-fried or grilled). Mezze is followed by a main meal and then fresh fruit or a sickly sweet dessert, such as baklavás (layers of filo pastry with honey and crushed nuts), halvás (made with semolina or sesame seeds), or loukoumi (Turkish delight). Travelling athletes should be able to find most of their usual foods in Greece. Two exceptions may be soy milk and tofu. Although the water in Greece is safe to drink, it is heavily chlorinated. Bottled water is inexpensive to buy and readily available.

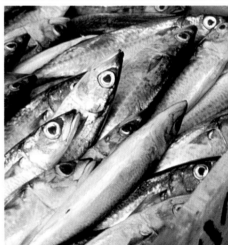

about the culture

Colourful, simple meals based on fresh seasonal produce, such as seafood, tomatoes, olives, eggplant, capsicum, artichokes, zucchini, okra, onion, garlic, melons, grapes, figs, oranges and lemons are a feature of Greek cuisine.

Typically, the first meal of the day is a strong coffee with sugar, followed by another at mid-morning! Greeks rarely eat breakfast – perhaps only a small cake or pastry. Lunch is usually more substantial and is eaten after 1pm. As in many other Mediterranean countries, shops and businesses close from 3pm to 5pm on most days for the infamous siesta. Dinner is eaten late in the evening, usually after 9pm.

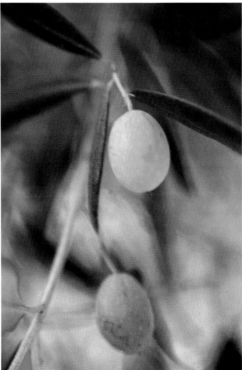

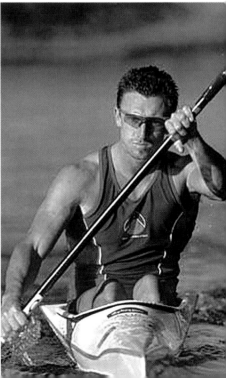

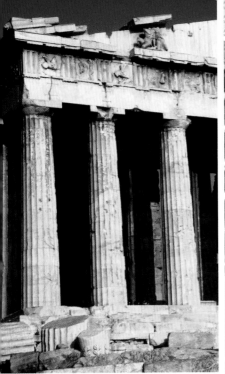

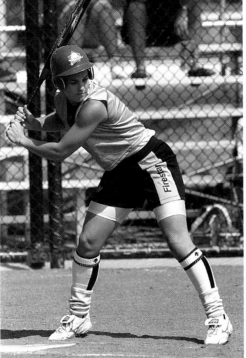

useful tip — sports foods

Sports drinks are available in powder and ready-to-drink forms from most supermarkets, though brands may be different to those at home. Cereal bars are sold in supermarkets and some corner stores, although choice is limited. Specialty sports products are more difficult to find. While bike, sports and health-food stores sell some products, they mainly consist of protein powders and body-building supplements. Usually, the safest bet is to bring cereal bars and sports products from home.

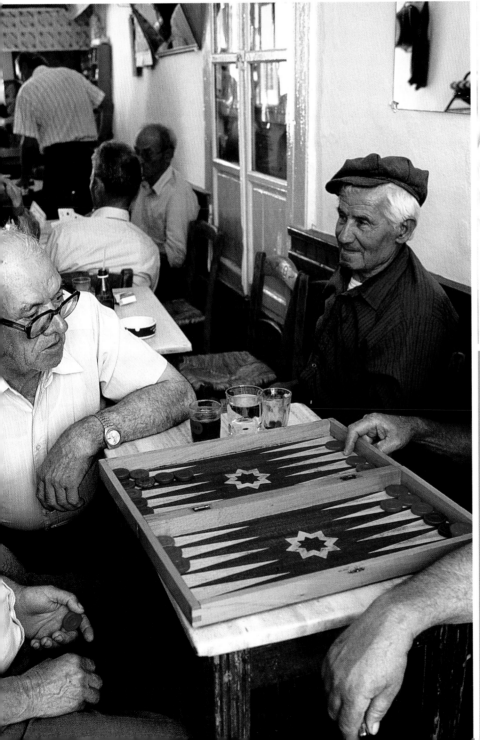

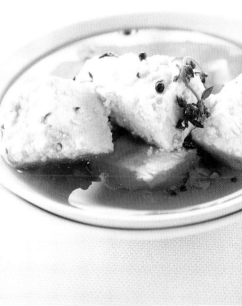

main nutrient sources

carbohydrate

Fresh bread, pita bread, crackers, pretzels, rice, pasta, potato, yogurt, rice pudding and seasonal fruit are widely available

protein

Seafood, lamb, kid, beef and poultry feature on most menus. Vegetarians should look for traditional dishes based on beans (e.g. lima beans, kidney beans, split peas) and lentils, or a vegetable omelette can often be whipped up on request

fat

Olive oil – few Greek dishes are made without it! Traditional Greek feta is delicious and features in many salads, pastries, sandwiches and mezze plates, but be aware that it is higher in fat than the Australian-made version.

greece

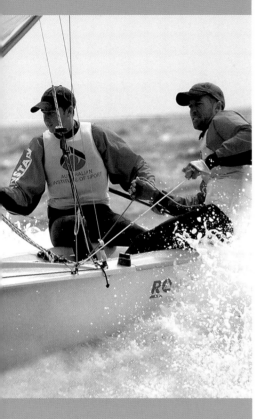

malcolm page and nathan wilmot — 470 sailing crew

"Athens is seriously hot, especially when we spend a lot of time in a concrete boat park. Good hydration is essential to keep us going all day long and sometimes into the night. Watch out for the olive oil in Athens — they add lots of it to everything."

lamb souvlaki with pita bread and tzatziki Serves 4-6

You will need 6-8 metal skewers or bamboo skewers, soaked in water
700g lamb, trimmed and
   cut into 3cm strips
1/4 cup lemon juice
1/2 tsp each salt and freshly
   ground pepper
1 1/2 tbs dried oregano
2 tsp minced garlic

1/4 cup grated onion
1 cup rice (omit for Low Fuel)
olive or canola oil spray
1 large white onion, thinly sliced
6-8 pita breads
2 cups shredded lettuce
200g cherry tomatoes, halved
1 Lebanese cucumber, diced
1 cup low-fat tzatziki dip

Place lamb in a non-metallic dish. Combine lemon juice, salt and pepper, 1 tbs of oregano, garlic and grated onion and pour over lamb. Cover and refrigerate for at least 2 hours (or overnight) to marinate. Cook rice according to packet instructions (omit for Low Fuel). Thread meat onto skewers. Preheat grill to medium-high heat. Grill skewers, turning occasionally, until brown on all sides. Meanwhile, spray a frypan with oil and cook sliced onion and remaining oregano over high heat, stirring occasionally, for 6 minutes or until soft and golden. Remove from pan. Quickly heat pita breads on grill until just warmed through, then split in half. Combine onion mixture and salad ingredients and divide between pita breads. Top with lamb and tzatziki, and serve with rice.

Analysis	High Fuel	Low Fuel
	4	6
energy (kj)	3015	1505
● protein (g)	53	33
● fat (g)	9	6
● CHO (g)	100	40
● iron		

vegetarian moussaka Serves 4-6 ✳

1 eggplant, sliced
olive or canola oil spray
1 onion, diced
1 tsp crushed garlic
1/2 red capsicum, deseeded and diced
2 zucchini, diced
6 button mushrooms, diced
440g can diced tomatoes
150g tomato paste
1 tbs soy sauce
1/2 tsp dried oregano
1/2 tsp dried basil

salt and freshly ground black pepper
375g low-fat ricotta cheese
150ml CARNATION Light & Creamy
   Evaporated Milk
5 potatoes, sliced and par-cooked
   (preferably steamed)
1/4 cup grated low-fat cheese
1/4 cup sliced sun-dried tomatoes
   (not in oil)
4 large or 6 small bread rolls
green salad, to serve

Preheat oven to 180°C (350°F) and grill or barbecue grill plate to medium-high heat. Lightly spray eggplant with oil and grill or barbecue, turning once, for 3-5 minutes or until cooked through. Set aside. Spray a frypan with oil and cook onion, garlic and capsicum over medium heat for 5 minutes or until soft. Add zucchini, mushrooms, tomatoes, tomato paste, soy sauce and herbs, season with salt and pepper, then simmer for 15 minutes or until the sauce thickens slightly. Combine ricotta cheese and milk in a bowl. Cover the base of a lasagne dish with a layer of potato slices, followed by a layer of eggplant, then a layer of vegetable mix. Repeat, then top with ricotta cheese mix. Sprinkle with grated cheese, then evenly place sun-dried tomatoes on top. Bake for 30-40 minutes or until golden brown. Serve with bread rolls and salad. **Option:** To make this a complete vegetarian meal, add 1/2 cup textured vegetable protein (TVP) mince to vegetable mixture. Add 1/4 cup water to re-hydrate TVP.

Analysis	High Fuel	Low Fuel
	4	6
energy (kj)	2877	1682
● protein (g)	34	21
● fat (g)	20	13
● CHO (g)	83	46
● calcium, vitamin C		

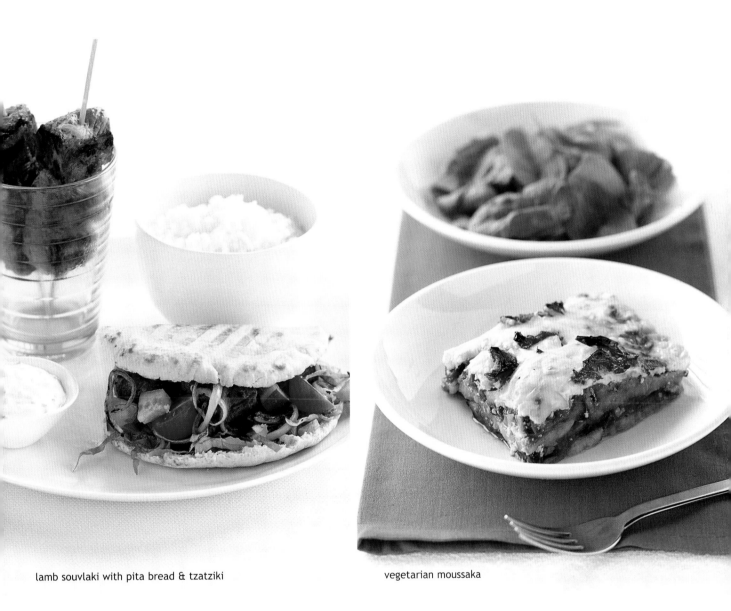

lamb souvlaki with pita bread & tzatziki

vegetarian moussaka

"Breakfast in many European countries is often full of meat. We always carry Vegemite with us. There is usually some type of bread available to make toast and sandwiches. It helps to keep things as similar as possible to our usual routine at home."

— robert newbery, diver

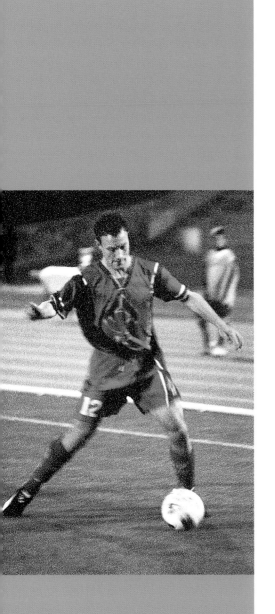

eli gilfedder —
soccer player

"When touring, I often find
that hotel buffets don't
provide much variety for
vegetarians. There are only
so many meals of pasta and
tomato sauce I can eat. Now,
when I travel, I make sure
to put in specific requests
ahead of time."

hummus Serves 4-6

olive or canola oil spray
1 small onion, finely chopped
1 tsp minced garlic
1 tsp ground cumin

2 tbs lemon juice
1/2 tsp paprika
425g can chickpeas,
    rinsed and drained

Analysis	High Fuel	Low Fuel
	4	6
energy (kj)	517	344
protein (g)	7	5
fat (g)	3	2
CHO (g)	15	10

Spray a non-stick frypan with oil and cook onion and
garlic over medium heat for 3-5 minutes or until soft.
Add cumin and cook for 1 minute. Process onion mixture
with remaining ingredients until smooth. Refrigerate
until required.

tzatziki Serves 4-6

2 Lebanese cucumbers, deseeded
    and chopped
200g PETERS FARM Natural
    No Fat Set Yogurt

1 tsp minced garlic
1/2 tsp ground cumin
1 tbs lemon juice

Analysis	High Fuel	Low Fuel
	4	6
energy (kj)	149	100
protein (g)	3	2
fat (g)	<1	<1
CHO (g)	4	3

Combine cucumbers, yogurt, garlic, cumin and lemon
juice. Refrigerate until required.

beetroot dip Serves 4-6

400g can beetroot balls, drained
1 tsp minced garlic
1 tsp ground coriander
2 tsp ground cumin

2 tsp lemon juice
200g PETERS FARM Natural
    No Fat Set Yogurt

Analysis	High Fuel	Low Fuel
	4	6
energy (kj)	307	205
protein (g)	4	3
fat (g)	<1	<1
CHO (g)	12	8

Combine beetroot, garlic, coriander, cumin, lemon juice
and yogurt. Process until roughly chopped. Refrigerate
until required.

eggplant dip Serves 4-6

500g eggplants
2 tsp minced garlic
1/2 onion, chopped
1 tbs lemon juice

2 tbs chopped fresh parsley
2 tbs olive oil
sea salt and freshly ground
    black pepper

Analysis	High Fuel	Low Fuel
	4	6
energy (kj)	480	320
protein (g)	2	1
fat (g)	10	6
CHO (g)	4	3

Preheat oven to 180°C (350°F). Bake eggplants for 45
minutes or until soft. Allow to cool slightly, peel and
discard skins. Roughly chop eggplants, place in a food
processor with remaining ingredients. Process until
smooth and creamy. Refrigerate until required.

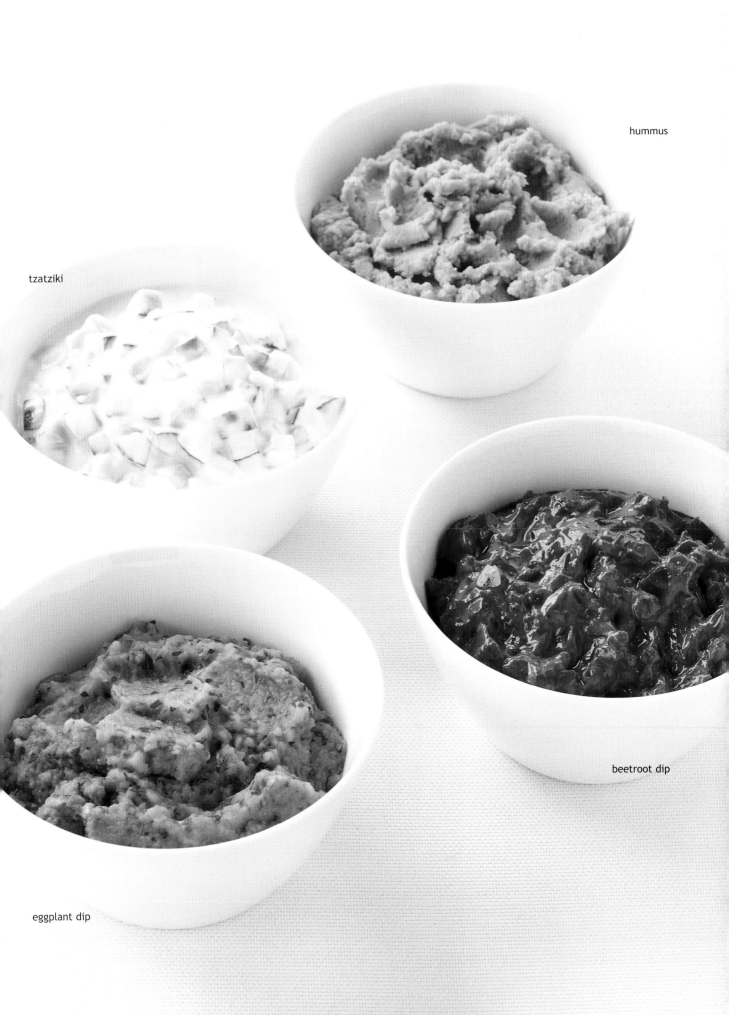

hummus

tzatziki

beetroot dip

eggplant dip

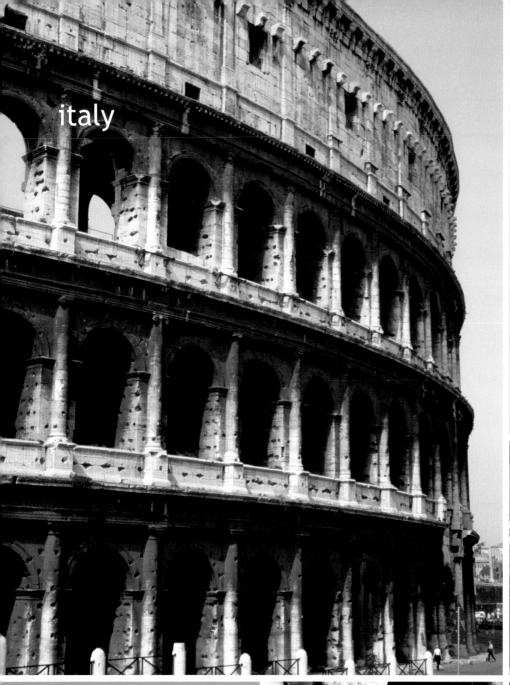

italy

food availability

A wide range of restaurants is available in larger metropolitan areas. Areas that cater for tourists will offer menus in English. Remember that pasta tends to be a small meal in Italy rather than the main-sized servings available in Australia. Pizzerias are abundant throughout Italy. Italian pizzas tend to have a flavoursome sauce and one or two simple toppings – don't expect to find a 'pizza with the lot'. Supermarkets 'supermercato' can be hard to find but streets of residential areas are usually littered with small grocery stores, which often have a better product range than you'd guess from their size. Many areas in Italy still observe a 'riposo' (mid-afternoon closing) from 1pm until 3:30-4pm.

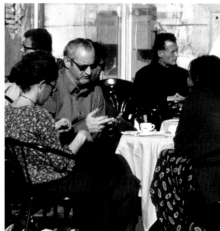

about the culture

Small quantities of meat, plenty of vegetables and legumes, sourdough bread, tomatoes, olive oil and wine are all elements of Italian cuisine that are thought to have a health-promoting effect. Italian specialties, such as pizza, pasta, frittata and bruschetta are familiar to most athletes, but authentic Italian cuisine can be very different to that served in the Italian eateries at home. Like many European cultures, Italians tend to enjoy a light breakfast – crusty bread dipped in milky coffee or coffee with bread, jam, cheese or sausage are popular choices. Lunch is traditionally the main meal of the day. It often begins with antipasto – an appetiser consisting of a variety of cold meats and pickled or preserved vegetables. A course of soup follows, then pasta or risotto and then a main course of meat or fish. Fresh fruit is a common dessert. Dinner tends to be a smaller meal of bread, cold meat and cheese or salad.

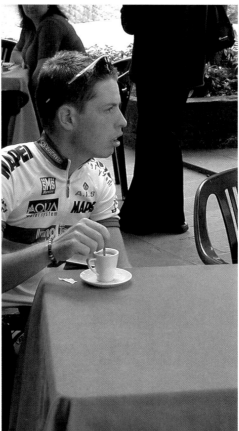

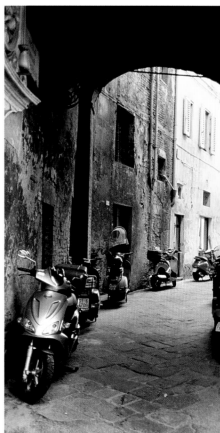

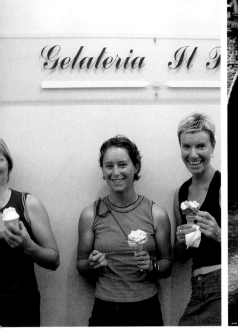

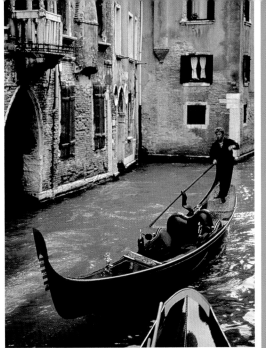

useful tips

▶ Gelato makes an excellent dessert choice, as it's fresh, light and available in a wide range of flavours
▶ Bakeries are everywhere in Italy. There are excellent choices to be made, but there are also many high-fat delights on offer
▶ Italians don't like to waste produce – every part of an animal is used in Italian dishes. It pays to learn some basic terminology or pack a phrase book if you want to avoid ordering ears, trotters, offal, sweetbreads and the like
▶ Italian bread is very crusty and requires much more chewing than Australian bread. This may cause you to eat less bread than usual. If you rely on bread for a large part of your carbohydrate intake, you may need to compensate by sourcing carbohydrate from other foods.

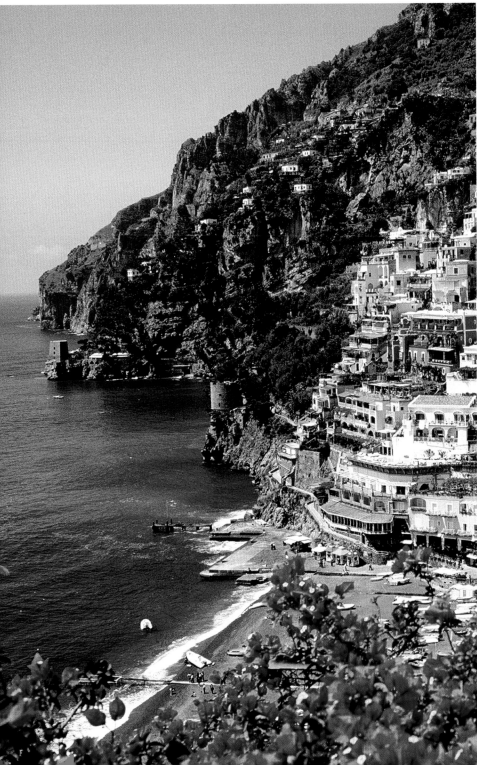

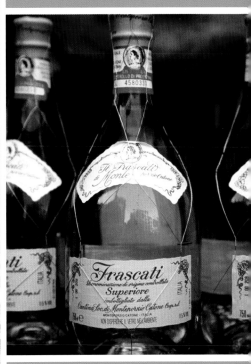

main nutrient sources

carbohydrate
Bread, rice, pasta, sweetened yogurt and fruit are widely available

protein
Veal, pork, poultry, cheese, eggs, yogurt and vegetarian sources, such as chickpeas and cannelini beans are all available

fat
Cream tends to be used more abundantly in northern Italy. Olive oil is a feature of many dishes and can cause the fat content of meals to be high.

italy

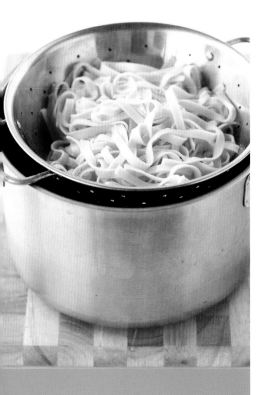

perfect pasta

▶ The key to cooking pasta is to use a large pan — pasta needs room to cook properly or it will stick together. As a basic guide, use 1 litre of water for every 100g of pasta and stir regularly.

▶ There is no need to add salt to the cooking water.

▶ Don't rinse pasta once it is drained — this will remove the starch, which helps your sauce to cling to the surface of the pasta.

tuna pasta bake Serves 4-6 ✳

1 each red, green and yellow capsicum
375-500g penne pasta
olive or canola oil spray
1 tsp minced garlic
6 green shallots, sliced
3 finger eggplants, sliced
1/4 cup balsamic vinegar

400g can tuna in brine, drained
250g low-fat cottage cheese
1 cup ultra-light sour cream (10% fat)
1/2 cup chopped fresh basil
freshly ground black pepper
1/4 cup grated parmesan cheese

Preheat grill to high. Place capsicums, skin-side up, under grill and cook for 8-10 minutes or until charred and blistered. Transfer to a heatproof bowl, cover with a plate or foil and set aside for 5 minutes (this helps to loosen the skin). Peel skin and slice flesh into strips. Preheat oven to 180°C (350°F). Cook pasta according to packet instructions, drain. Meanwhile, spray a non-stick saucepan with oil and cook garlic and green shallots over medium heat for 3 minutes or until soft. Add eggplant and vinegar and cook for a further 3-5 minutes or until soft. Combine capsicum, pasta and eggplant mixture with tuna, cottage cheese, sour cream, basil and pepper and transfer to an ovenproof dish or 4 individual dishes. Sprinkle with parmesan and bake for 15 minutes or until golden brown.

Analysis	High Fuel	Low Fuel
	4	6
energy (kj)	2991	1699
protein (g)	50	31
fat (g)	14	9
CHO (g)	93	48
vitamin C		

pasta with chicken and corn Serves 4-6 ✳

300-375g spiral pasta
olive or canola oil spray
1 tsp minced garlic
6 green shallots, chopped
400-500g chicken breast fillets, sliced

150g button mushrooms, sliced
300-400g can creamed corn
100g sun-dried tomatoes (not in oil)
1/2 cup MAGGI Real Chicken Stock
1/2 cup ultra-light sour cream (10% fat)

Cook pasta according to packet instructions. Meanwhile, spray a non-stick frypan with oil and cook garlic, green shallots, chicken and mushrooms over medium-high heat for 15 minutes or until chicken is tender and cooked through. Add corn, sun-dried tomatoes and stock and simmer for 5 minutes. Remove from heat and stir through sour cream. Stir pasta through sauce and serve immediately.

Analysis	High Fuel	Low Fuel
	4	6
energy (kj)	2916	1611
protein (g)	45	24
fat (g)	14	8
CHO (g)	91	50
vitamin C		

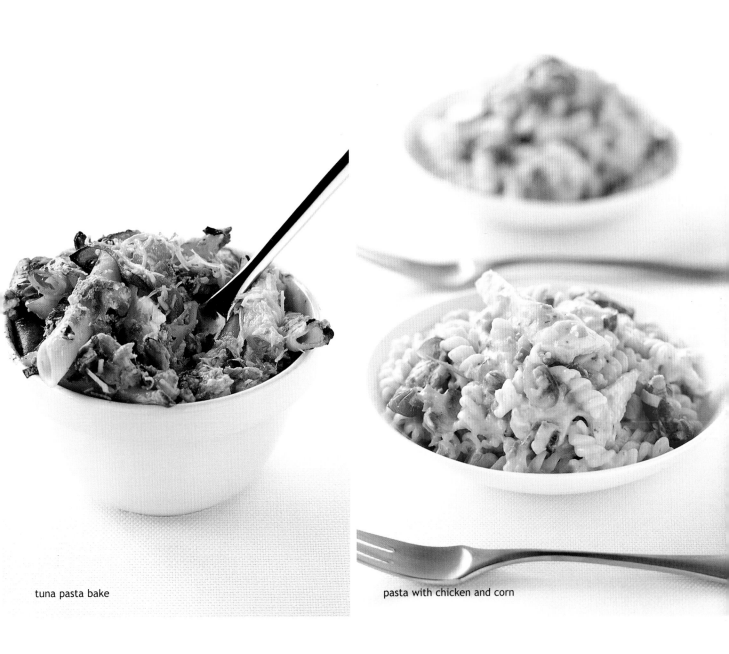

tuna pasta bake

pasta with chicken and corn

"I have mainly travelled through Austria and Italy, and I have learned to be prepared for different foods. For two months straight, all we had were bread rolls with a selection of meats, cheeses and jams for breakfast. You can never beat Vegemite on toast but most hotels don't understand the concept of toast at all."

— toby kane, paralympic alpine skier

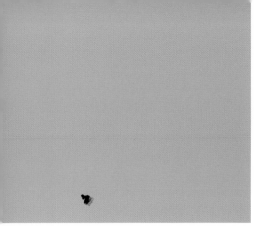

gnocchi with pumpkin sauce and cheese bread   Serves 4-6 ✻

700g potato gnocchi
250g cherry tomatoes, halved
freshly ground black pepper
olive or canola oil spray
1 leek (white part only), sliced
500g pumpkin, peeled, deseeded
   and chopped
1 cup vegetable stock
150ml CARNATION Light & Creamy
   Evaporated Milk

150g baby spinach
1 tbs chopped fresh sage

cheese bread:
6-8 large slices sourdough bread
1-2 cloves garlic
3/4-1 cup grated parmesan cheese

Cook gnocchi according to packet instructions. Preheat oven to 200°C (400°F). Arrange tomatoes, cut-side up, on an oven tray lined with non-stick paper. Season with pepper. Bake for 10-15 minutes or until just soft. Meanwhile, spray a non-stick saucepan with oil and cook leek over medium heat for 3-5 minutes or until soft. Add pumpkin and stock and simmer for 3 minutes or until pumpkin is soft. Add milk and process or blend until smooth. Return mixture to pan, add spinach and heat until wilted. Stir through sage and tomatoes. Season with pepper. Add gnocchi and toss to combine. Meanwhile, to make cheese bread, toast bread under grill. Slice garlic in half and rub over warm bread. Sprinkle with cheese and return to grill until cheese is slightly melted. Serve gnocchi with cheese bread.

Analysis	High Fuel	Low Fuel
	4	6
energy (kj)	2507	1485
● protein (g)	30	17
● fat (g)	11	6
● CHO (g)	90	55
● calcium, vitamin C		

ham & zucchini risotto   Serves 4-6

olive or canola oil spray
1 leek (white part only), sliced
1 tsp minced garlic
2 sticks celery, sliced
200g chopped ham
1 1/2-2 cups arborio rice
875ml-1 litre MAGGI Real
   Chicken Stock

200-375ml CARNATION Light
   & Creamy Evaporated Milk
3 small zucchini, sliced
1 cup frozen peas
2 tbs chopped fresh parsley
1/3 cup grated parmesan cheese
freshly ground black pepper

Spray a non-stick saucepan with oil and cook leek, garlic, celery and ham over medium heat for 3-5 minutes or until leek is soft. Add rice and cook, stirring, for 1 minute or until rice is coated. Add stock and milk and bring to the boil. Simmer, stirring occasionally, for 20 minutes or until the rice is soft. Add zucchini and peas and cook for a further 5 minutes. Remove from heat and stir through parsley, cheese and pepper.

Analysis	High Fuel	Low Fuel
	4	6
energy (kj)	2639	1428
● protein (g)	34	20
● fat (g)	9	6
● CHO (g)	100	50
● calcium, iron		

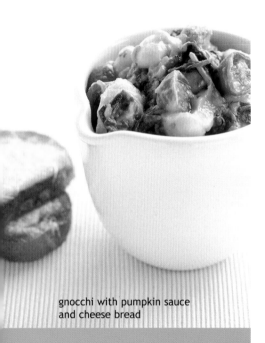

gnocchi with pumpkin sauce
and cheese bread

knock-out gnocchi

▸ Cook gnocchi until it floats to the surface of the pan, then cook for 1 minute more — it will start breaking up if left for any longer than this. Serve immediately, otherwise the high starch content will begin to dull the flavour.

▸ Gnocchi can be served with a variety of sauces.

▸ Gnocchi is also delicious when served in a salad with rocket and parmesan.

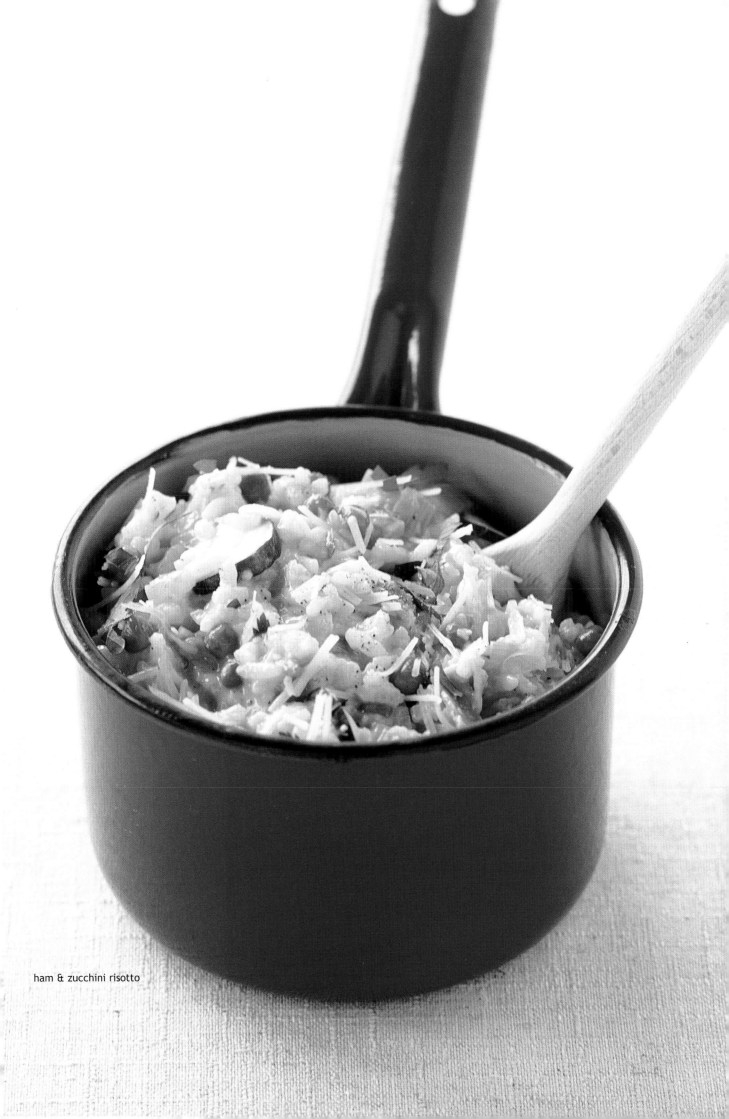

ham & zucchini risotto

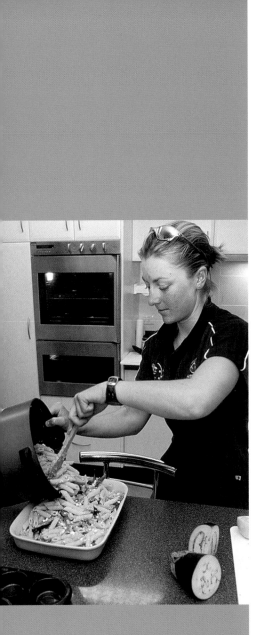

chocolate bread Serves 6-8 ✳

500g plain flour, plus extra for dusting
2 x 7g sachets dried yeast
2 tsp salt

2 tbs caster sugar
1/2 cup chocolate hazelnut spread
milk, to brush

Combine flour, yeast, salt and sugar in a large bowl. Make a well in the centre and add 11/2 cups warm water, a little at a time, mixing until a soft dough forms. Turn dough onto a floured surface and knead for a few minutes, until dough is soft and elastic. Dust the bowl with flour. Shape dough into a ball, return it to the bowl and cover with a tea towel. Place in a warm spot (such as a sunny room or an oven that has been heated briefly and turned off) for about 40 minutes or until dough has doubled in size. Punch air out of dough and turn out onto a floured surface. Use a rolling pin to roll dough into a rectangle about 5mm thick. Heat hazelnut spread in microwave on MEDIUM heat for 25 seconds, then spread over dough, leaving a 2cm border around the edges. Starting at one of the longer sides of the rectangle, roll dough up to form a long cylinder shape, then roll cylinder to form a snail shell. Place dough on a tray lined with baking paper and leave to rise in a warm spot for about 1 hour. Brush the top with a little milk and transfer to a cold oven, set at 180°C (350°F) and bake for 25 minutes or until bread is golden on top.

Analysis	High Fuel	Low Fuel
	6	8
energy (kj)	1772	1329
protein (g)	10	8
fat (g)	8	6
● CHO (g)	77	58

lemon gelati Serves 4-6 ✳

1 cup caster sugar
1/2 cup lemon juice, strained
2 eggwhites, lightly beaten

blueberries and strawberries,
    to serve (optional)
biscotti, to serve (optional)

Heat sugar and 2 cups water in a small saucepan over low heat, stirring, for 5 minutes or until sugar dissolves. Bring to the boil and simmer, uncovered, for 10 minutes or until syrupy. Remove from heat and allow to cool. Stir in lemon juice. Pour mixture into a slice pan and place in freezer until just frozen. Transfer to a food processor or bowl, add eggwhites and process or beat with an electric mixer until combined. Return to pan and refreeze until just frozen. Process or beat mixture again, then refreeze until firm. Serve with berries and biscotti, if desired.

Analysis	High Fuel	Low Fuel
	4	6
energy (kj)	1049	700
protein (g)	3	2
● fat (g)	<1	<1
● CHO (g)	60	40
● vitamin C		

naomi williams — cyclist

"Being based with the Australian Women's Road Cycling team in a little town in Italy for 6-7 months of the year has certainly influenced my cooking skills. We cook with lots of the local foods — olive oil, balsamic vinegar and parmesan cheese. We even get to buy some of those foods straight from the farms or little factories where they are produced. At some of the races, they give food for prizes — pasta, sauces, once we won a whole pig! All the prizes end up in our recipes."

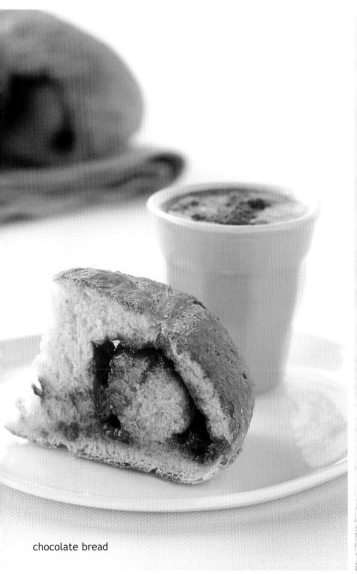

chocolate bread

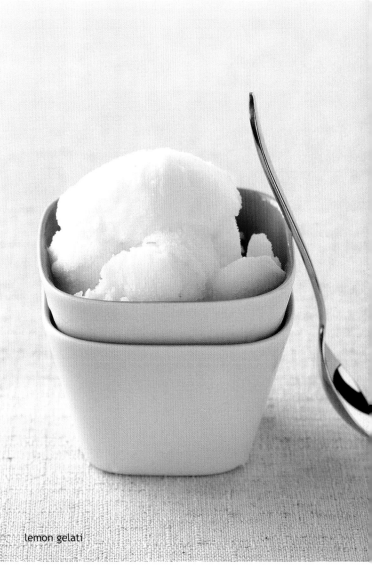

lemon gelati

"After watching the AIS men's U/23 road cyclists tackle my cooking classes, I wondered how they would ever manage to become totally self-sufficient during their six month stint in rural Italy, but being thrown in at the deep end worked. Visiting a few months later, I saw that they had not only survived, but thrived. In fact, they gave me a lesson on how to bake fresh bread. Of course, I had to get their chocolate bread recipe for this book."

— louise burke, head of department of sports nutrition, AIS

france

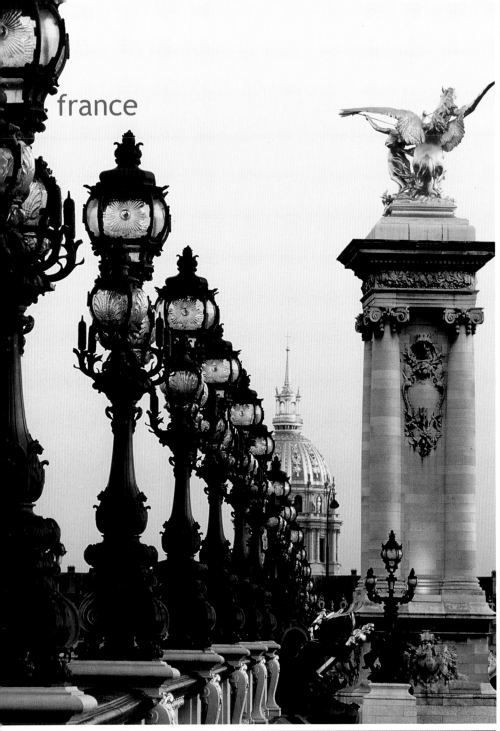

food availability

In larger metropolitan areas, travelling athletes will find all the usual food franchises and fast-food outlets, and will be able to choose from a variety of cuisines. Smaller towns have at least one restaurant or bar providing more traditional meals, such as steak frites (steak and chips), poulet rôti (roast chicken) and salade niçoise (salad with tuna, potato or rice and olives). Bread is almost always complimentary in French restaurants and is supplied as often as it is needed during a meal. Most foods can be found in France, although some Asian foods, such as curry pastes and sauces may be difficult to find in smaller locations. Milk in France is usually UHT and found on the supermarket shelf rather than in the fridge. Markets are a feature of French culture and each region holds at least one per week – these are a great source of fresh produce. A limited selection of breakfast cereals is likely to be available (it may pay to take your own). Cereal bars tend to be smaller than products available in Australia and are often chocolate coated. Sports stores, such as Decathlon, stock a good range of sports drinks, bars, powders and gels.

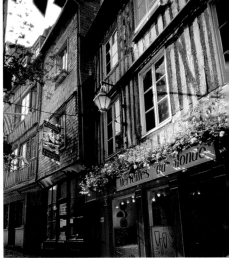

about the culture

While goose fat, duck's fat, butter, cream and cheese feature in many French recipes, the cuisine is extremely diverse. The French have access to an abundance of good-quality fruit, vegetables, seafood, meat and poultry. Although renowned for haute cuisine, they are also skilled at making simple, delicious meals out of produce in peak season. French breakfasts usually consist of coffee or hot chocolate with pastry or bread and jam. Lunch is the main meal of the day and is traditionally a 3-4 course affair. Businesses typically close for a 2-hour break to allow people time to enjoy their lunch. Dinner tends to be a lighter meal of bread, cold meat and cheese or salad. In France, snacking is generally only for children.

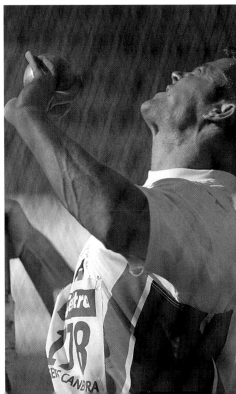

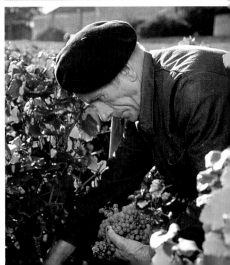

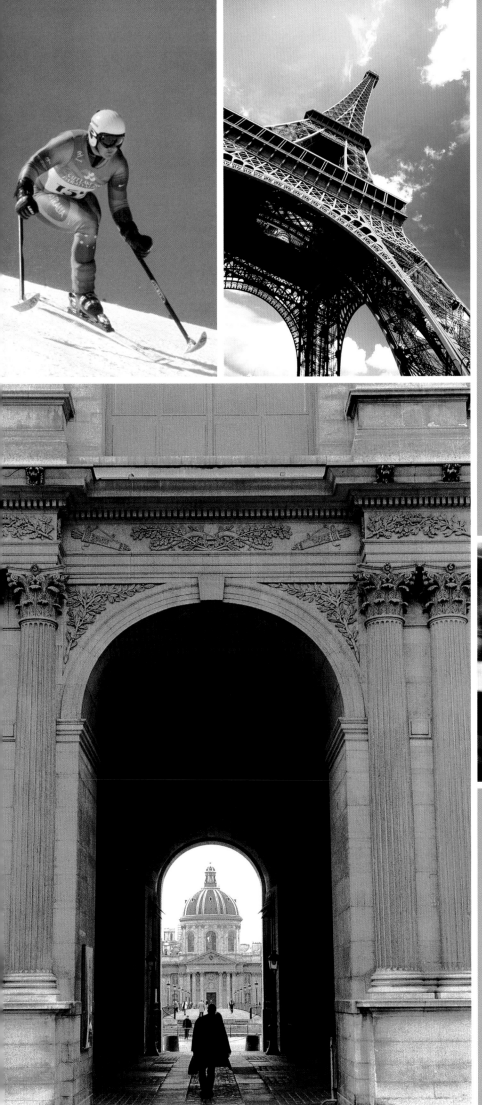

useful tips

▶ The French hold their thumb up (rather than their index finger) to indicate '1'. Even if your pronunciation is perfect, use your thumb or be prepared to be given two of everything you ask for

▶ Filled baguettes and sandwiches are widely available in France. In smaller locations, sandwiches are often limited to 'jambon' (ham), 'fromage' (cheese) or a 'super sandwich' (ham and cheese). 'Salade' on a menu board means lettuce, not a selection of salad ingredients. Cheese sandwiches typically include a thick spread of butter, plus slabs of a selection of high-fat cheeses

▶ It is rare to find the snack-laden kiosks that are typical of Australian sporting venues. Be prepared and take your own food supplies

▶ Vegetarian choices are not regularly available in France. Goose and pig's fat are commonly used as cooking fats. Foods such as French fries, which are commonly cooked in vegetable oil in Australia, may not be vegetarian choices in France.

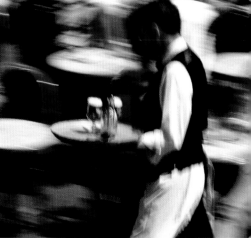

main nutrient sources

carbohydrate
Bread, rice, pasta, potato, sweetened yogurt and fruit are widely available

protein
Meat, fish, poultry and dairy will feature on menus. You may also find some unusual sources of protein, such as boar, various types of offal and goat. Vegetarian sources of protein may be difficult to obtain

fat
Rich sauces, high-fat cheeses, full-cream dairy products and animal-based cooking fats are all features of French cuisine.

france

vegetarian quiche Serves 4-6

olive or canola oil spray
1 sheet frozen reduced-fat puff
  pastry, thawed
3 eggs
1 cup CARNATION Light & Creamy
  Evaporated Milk
salt and freshly ground black pepper,
  to taste
$1/2$ cup broccoli florets

$1/2$ red capsicum, deseeded and diced
1 tomato, diced
1 onion, diced
4 button mushrooms, sliced
2 vegetarian sausages, sliced
  (optional)
$1/4$ cup grated low-fat cheese
4 large or 6 small bread rolls
tossed salad, to serve (optional)

Preheat oven to 180°C (350°F). Lightly spray a 20cm pie dish with oil and line with pastry (stretch pastry up edge of dish). Mix eggs, milk, salt and pepper in a bowl, then add broccoli, capsicum, tomato and onion. Pour mixture into pie dish and arrange mushrooms and vegetarian sausage, if desired, over the top. Sprinkle with cheese and bake for 30 minutes or until egg mixture has set. Serve with bread rolls and a tossed salad.

Analysis	High Fuel	Low Fuel
	4	6
energy (kj)	2456	1645
● protein (g)	30	21
● fat (g)	21	14
● CHO (g)	66	44
● calcium, vitamin C		

niçoise salad Serves 4-6

12 small chat potatoes, halved
150g baby spinach
1 cup halved cherry tomatoes
200g baby green beans, trimmed
  and blanched
400g can tuna in brine, drained
8 pitted black olives, halved
$1/3$ cup fresh basil leaves

4 hard-boiled eggs, peeled
  and quartered
$1/4$ cup low-fat mayonnaise
1 tbs Dijon mustard
2 tsp lemon juice
freshly ground black pepper
4 large or 6 small bread rolls

Analysis	High Fuel	Low Fuel
	4	6
energy (kj)	2863	1672
● protein (g)	49	31
○ fat (g)	15	9
○ CHO (g)	81	44
● iron, vitamin C		

Boil potatoes in a saucepan for 8-10 minutes or until cooked. Drain. Combine spinach, tomatoes, beans and potatoes in a large serving bowl. Flake tuna over the top and scatter with olives, basil and eggs. Combine mayonnaise, mustard and lemon juice and drizzle over salad. Season with pepper. Serve with bread rolls.

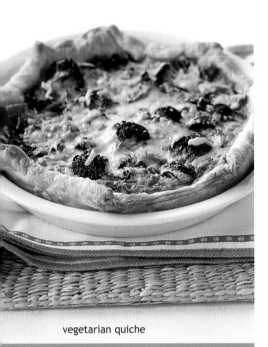

vegetarian quiche

golden puff pastry

▶ Before lining a dish with puff pastry, lightly grease the dish with oil spray so it won't stick. Once the puff pastry is in place, return to the freezer for 10 minutes — this will make the pastry solid and will prevent it from shrinking in the oven.

▶ If you want your pastry to have a crisp base, place a metal tray in the oven while preheating, then place your dish on top — the metal tray will generate enough heat to cook the base through.

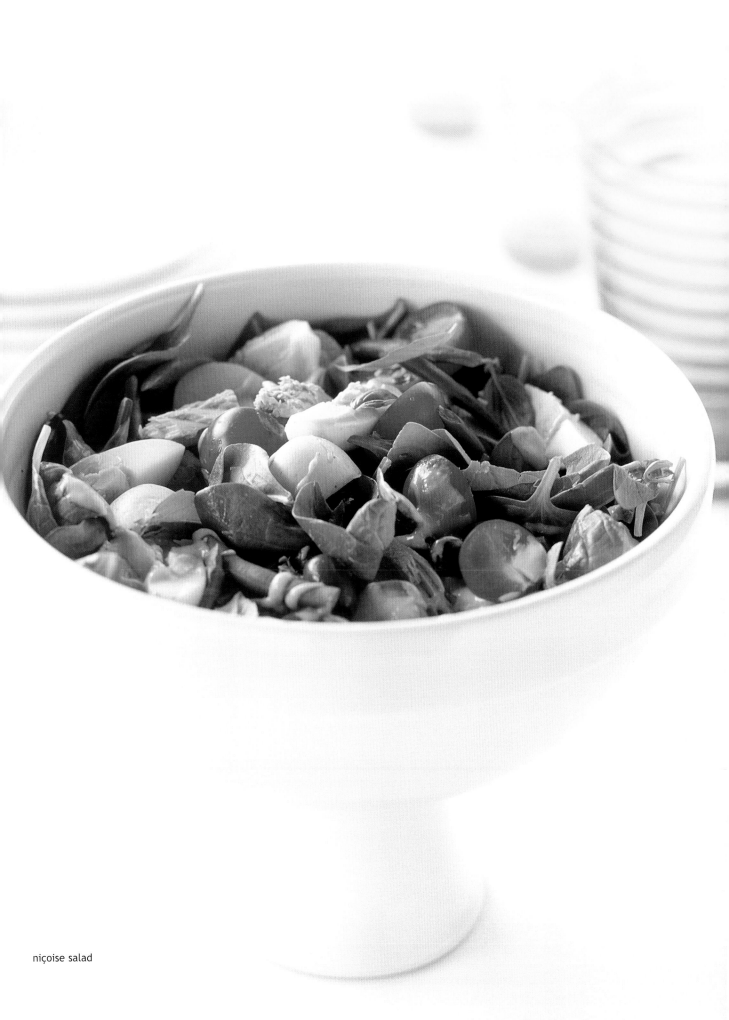

niçoise salad

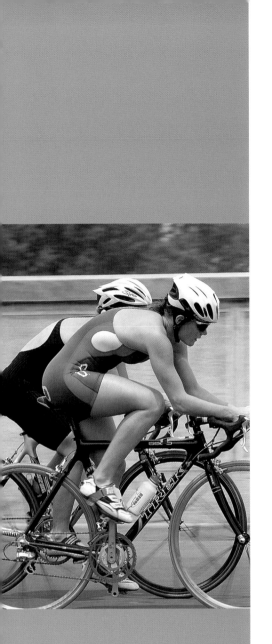

nikki egyed — triathlete

"Our European training base is in the Savoie region of France, an area famous for 'fromage' — that's cheese! I like cheese but it's hard to perform well when eating it at every meal. Fortunately, our dietitian convinced the chefs to vary the menu."

french crepes with berries Serves 4-6 ✻

150g blueberries
150g strawberries, hulled and halved
4 tbs caster sugar
1 vanilla bean, split lengthways or
    1 tsp vanilla essence
2 tsp cornflour
70g plain flour

20g butter or canola margarine, melted
1 tsp lemon zest
2 eggs
3/4 cup skim milk
olive or canola oil spray
4-6 scoops PETERS Light & Creamy
    Vanilla Ice-cream (optional)

Heat berries, 3 tablespoons sugar, vanilla bean/essence and 300ml water in a saucepan over low heat for 5 minutes or until sugar dissolves. Mix cornflour with 1 tablespoon water and stir into berry mixture. Simmer, stirring constantly, for 2 minutes or until sauce thickens, then cover and remove from heat. Sift flour into a bowl, then stir in remaining sugar and make a well in the centre. Combine butter/margarine, lemon zest, eggs and milk in a small jug. Whisk into dry ingredients and stir until mixture resembles a smooth batter. Lightly spray a small non-stick frypan with oil, add 2-3 tablespoons of batter to pan and tilt pan so it covers the base. Cook over medium heat for 2 minutes or until golden underneath. Flip and cook the other side until golden. Remove from pan and transfer to a low oven to keep warm while you cook remaining crepes. Serve with sauce and a scoop of ice-cream, if desired.

Analysis	High Fuel	Low Fuel
	4	6
energy (kj)	1302	869
protein (g)	10	7
● fat (g)	9	6
● CHO (g)	48	32

low-fat crème brûlée Serves 4

170g pitted dates, halved
100ml golden syrup
1 vanilla bean, split lengthways,
    or 1 tsp vanilla essence

1 litre NESTLÉ All Natural 99%
    Fat Free Vanilla Yogurt
1 cup white sugar

Cook dates, golden syrup and vanilla bean/essence in a small saucepan over medium heat for 5 minutes or until dates are soft. Divide mixture between four 1-cup capacity ramekins or glasses. Spoon yogurt over the top. Stir sugar and 1/2 cup water in a saucepan over low heat until sugar dissolves. Bring to the boil and cook over high heat for 5-10 minutes or until sugar turns dark golden. Immediately remove from heat and pour a thin layer of caramel over yogurt. Allow to set and serve immediately.

Analysis	4 serves
energy (kj)	2587
protein (g)	16
● fat (g)	<1
● CHO (g)	137
● calcium	

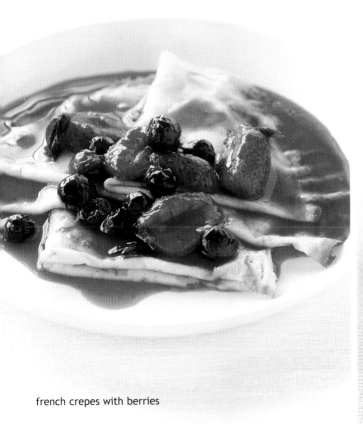

french crepes with berries

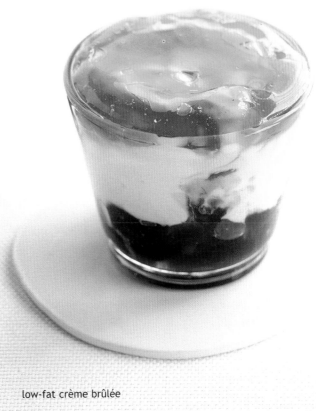

low-fat crème brûlée

"I know a lot of athletes have horror travel stories, but you really can't beat the food at our yearly training camp in St Moritz, Switzerland. It is an incentive to get on the team — the bircher muesli is fantastic."

— liz kell, rower

asia

An intriguing melting pot of cultures, Asia explodes with imagery and flavours that will remain with you forever. From the refined and minimal fare of Japan to the fragrant dishes of Vietnam and Thailand and the hot and spicy tastes of India, you are destined to love the contrast and balance struck so uniquely by each country.

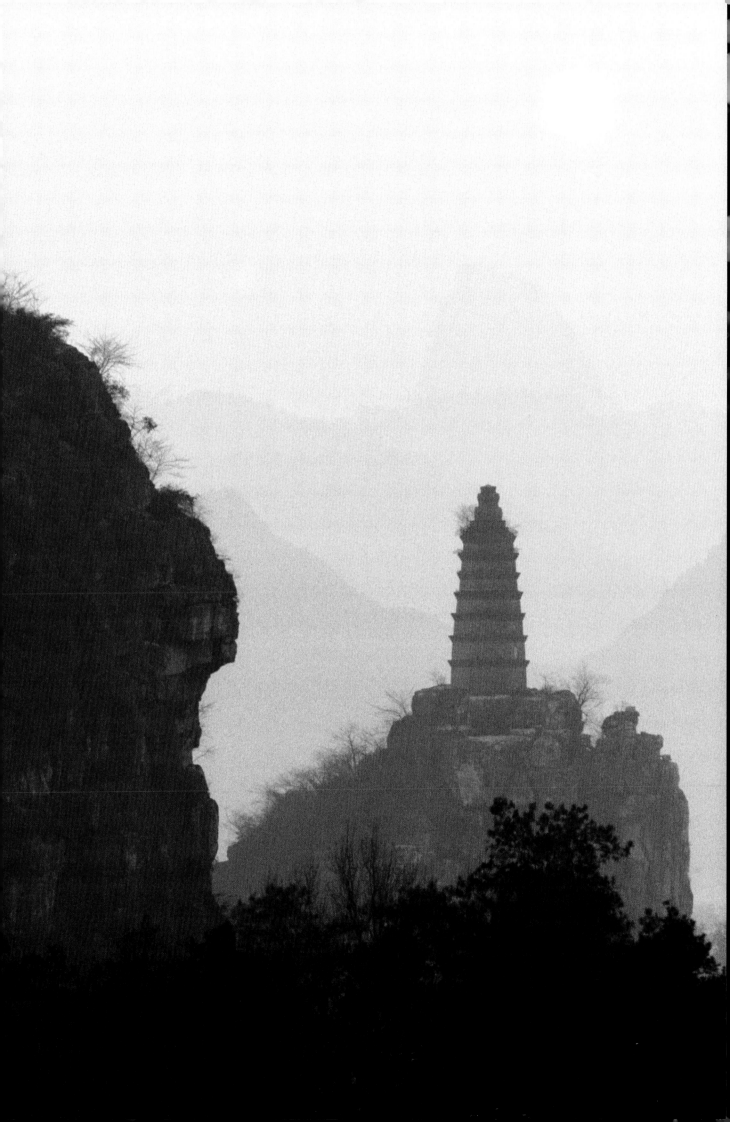

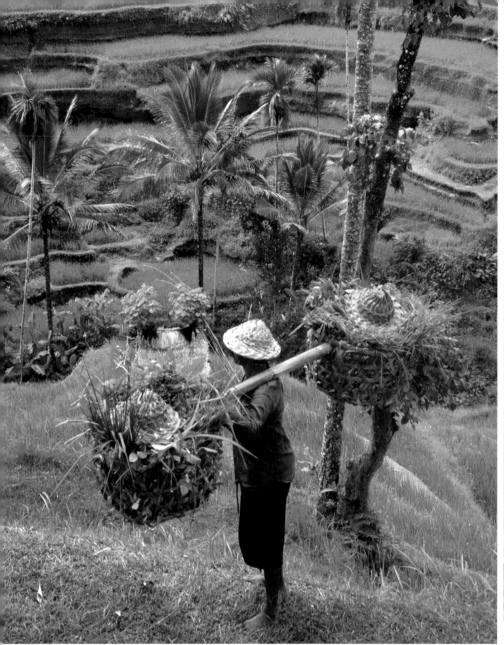

food availability

Food is very inexpensive in most Asian countries – the exception being Japan. There is a large range of restaurant styles to visit, from local traditional types to Western-style restaurants. However, travelling athletes should be aware of the potentially poor hygiene of some of the local establishments. If you are tempted by the abundant seafood available in much of Asia, it is important to choose a reputable restaurant as seafood is a major source of food poisoning in the region. Food availability varies according to the country of travel. More developed locations will have well-stocked supermarkets with a range of familiar foods. In less-developed areas, street markets are the major source of food and Western produce can be difficult to obtain. In this situation, it is more practical to rely on restaurants than attempt to self-cater. Dairy products, breakfast cereals, cereal bars and special sports products can be hard to find in Asia, so it is useful to take supplies from home.

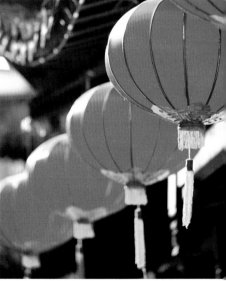

about the culture

Asian cuisine varies from the fresh, light food of Japan, to the fragrant food of Vietnam and Thailand, to the hot, spicy food of India. The one factor common to all is that rice or noodles are eaten with virtually every meal. Fresh ingredients are a priority, vegetables are easy to obtain and meat servings tend to be small. Authentic Asian food is usually very different to that provided in Western restaurants. In many Asian countries, breakfast is likely to consist of a savoury broth, noodles or a sweet steamed bun filled with savoury ingredients. Major hotels will provide Western breakfast choices but they tend to be influenced by American culture, with donuts and coffee being regular features. Traditionally, lunch and dinner are eaten at home and consist of 4-5 different dishes that are shared among a family. However, as street vendors are prolific throughout Asia it is also acceptable to grab a quick meal on the street.

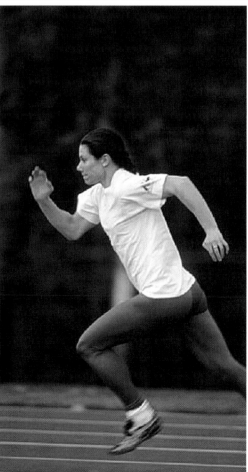

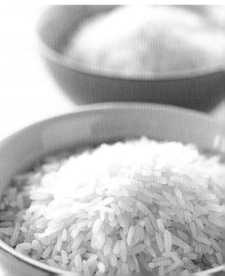

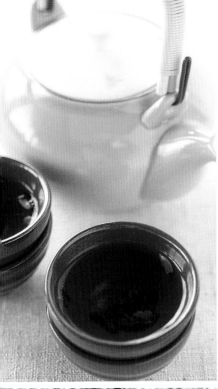

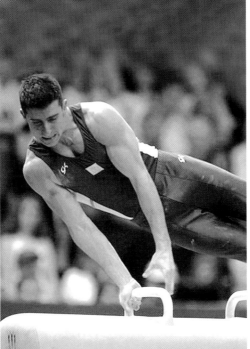

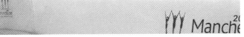

useful tips

▶ Consuming sufficient protein, vitamins and minerals can be difficult, especially when food hygiene is poor. A liquid meal supplement is an essential item to take to Asia

▶ Asian bread tends to be sweeter and lower in fibre than bread in Australia. The availability of high-fibre cereals is also limited. To avoid constipation, eat plenty of fresh fruit and vegetables, and take some cereal, cereal bars and dried fruit from home

▶ Food safety is a major issue in many Asian countries – always adopt conservative behaviour regarding food hygiene.

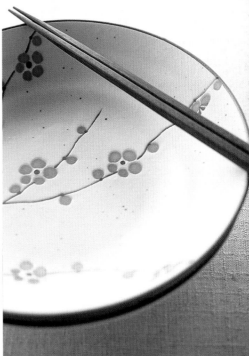

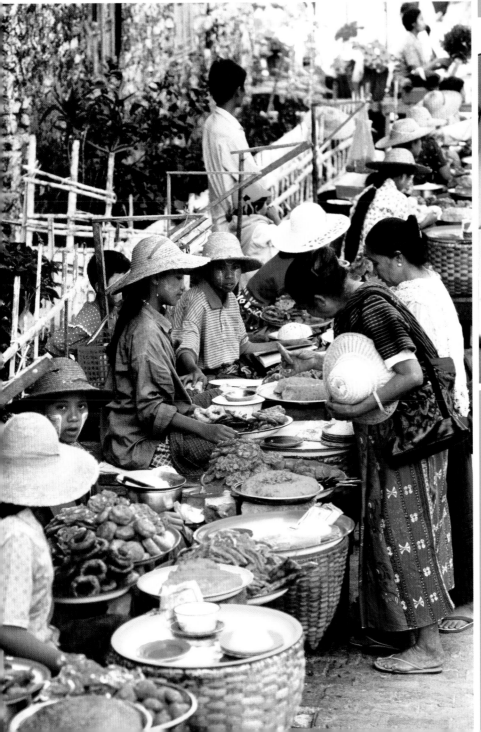

main nutrient sources

carbohydrate

Rice and noodles will be found everywhere, plus baguettes in Vietnam, flat breads (such as *chapatti*) in India, and fresh fruit and juice in tropical areas

protein

Meat, fish, poultry and eggs will be found in most areas, however the quality of cuts may differ significantly from those available in Australia. Dairy is uncommon in these parts

fat

Fatty meats are highly valued throughout much of Asia and deep-fried foods are common. The rich coconut-based curries are also high in fat.

asia

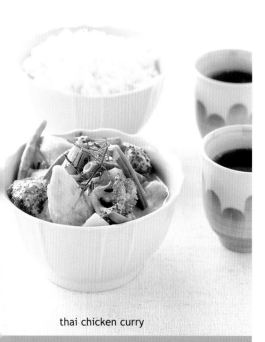

thai chicken curry

tempting thai curries

▶ Contrary to popular belief, green curries are generally hotter than red curries. If you don't like your curry too hot, start with a small amount of curry paste and then add more as you go.

▶ If your curry does become too hot, add sugar to temper the heat.

▶ For a no-fail curry seasoning, combine equal amounts of fish sauce and palm sugar or brown sugar — start with 1-2 tablespoons of each.

thai chicken curry   Serves 4-6 ✳

1-1½ cups jasmine rice
olive or canola oil spray
500g chicken breast fillets, sliced
1-2 tbs green curry paste
375ml can CARNATION Light & Creamy Evaporated Milk
1 tsp coconut essence
4 kaffir lime leaves, finely shredded, plus extra, to garnish

200g green beans, trimmed and halved
200g baby corn
200g broccoli florets
200g can bamboo shoots, rinsed and drained
2 tbs MAGGI Fish Sauce
2 tbs brown sugar
1 tbs cornflour

Steam rice according to packet instructions. Spray a non-stick wok with oil and stirfry chicken over medium-high heat for 5 minutes or until browned. Add curry paste and stirfry until fragrant. Stir in milk, coconut essence and lime leaves and bring to the boil. Reduce heat to low, add beans, corn, broccoli and bamboo shoots and simmer for 5 minutes or until beans are tender. Add fish sauce and brown sugar. Blend cornflour with 2 tablespoons water, stir into wok and cook, stirring, until curry boils and thickens slightly. Garnish with extra lime leaves and serve with rice.

Analysis	High Fuel	Low Fuel
	4	6
energy (kj)	2877	1666
● protein (g)	47	30
● fat (g)	13	8
● CHO (g)	92	48
● calcium, iron, vitamin C		

sushi   Serves 4-6

2 cups sushi rice
¼ cup seasoned rice vinegar
2 tbs caster sugar
2 eggs, beaten
6 sheets nori
wasabi paste, to taste, plus extra, to serve (optional)
1 Lebanese cucumber, deseeded and cut into long strips

1 red capsicum, deseeded and cut into long strips
1 small carrot, peeled and cut into long strips
200g smoked salmon, cut into long strips
50g pickled ginger, drained (optional)
½ cup soy sauce, to serve

Place rice in a microwave steamer with 3 cups boiling water. Secure lid and heat in microwave on HIGH for 5 minutes. Stir, then heat on MEDIUM for 10 minutes. Add rice vinegar and sugar and stir well. Spread over a large baking tray and allow to cool. Meanwhile, cook eggs in a non-stick frypan for 2-3 minutes or until set. Remove from pan and cut into long strips. Place 1 sheet of nori, rough-side up, on a bamboo sushi mat or tea towel. With wet fingers, spread one-sixth of rice over nori. Cover nori all the way to the edges, except for a 4cm strip on the far side. Press rice down firmly. Spread a small amount of wasabi along the centre of rice, if desired. Place strips of cucumber, capsicum, carrot, salmon, egg and ginger, if desired, across the centre. Starting at the edge closest to you, use the mat or tea towel to roll sushi into a log. Press firmly as you roll. Dip a knife in water and slice log into 6 pieces. Repeat with remaining ingredients. Serve with soy sauce for dipping and extra wasabi, if desired.

Option: Salmon can be substituted with strips of tofu.

Analysis	High Fuel	Low Fuel
	4	6
energy (kj)	2579	1719
● protein (g)	33	22
● fat (g)	6	4
● CHO (g)	105	70
● vitamin C		

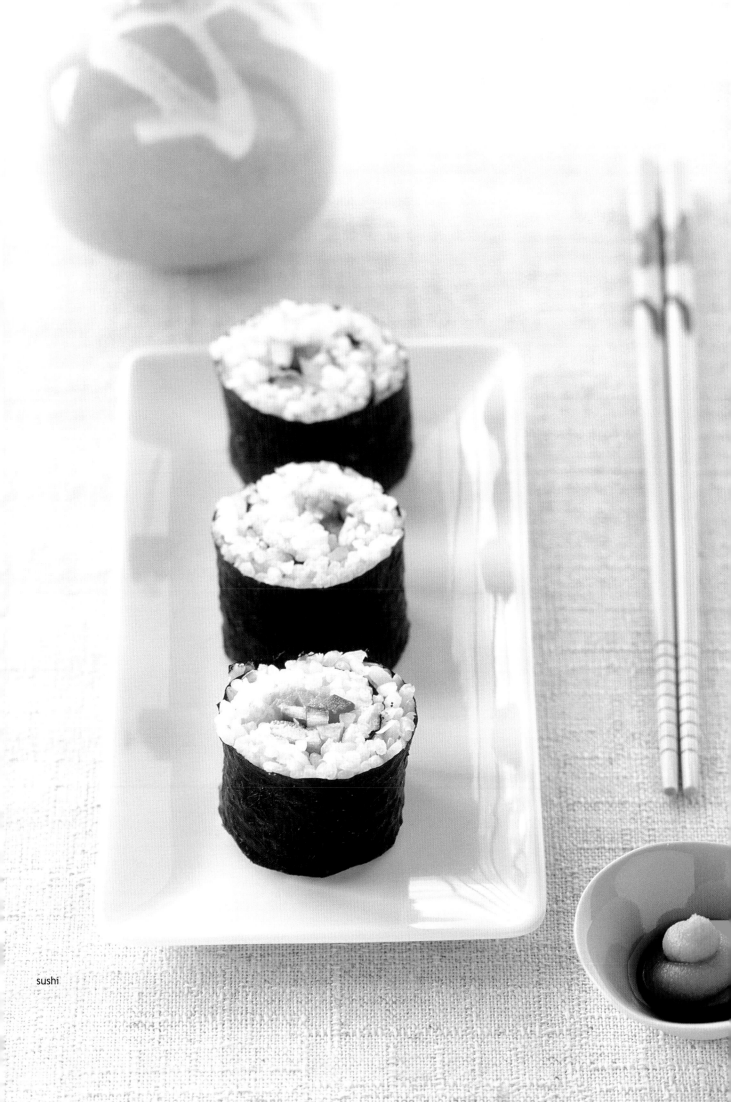

sushi

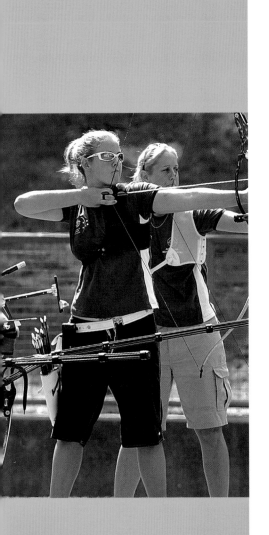

jo-ann galbraith — archer

"When travelling in Asia, be prepared to try anything. You may be served sea cucumbers, but you may also discover some great dishes, such as pull goki. This is marinated lamb or beef that is cooked on a Korean barbecue, then wrapped in a leaf with chilli, garlic and rice. I would never have discovered this great dish if I hadn't been prepared to jump in and try new things."

chilli beef with choy sum Serves 4-6

1-2 cups rice
2 tbs MAGGI Oyster Sauce
2 tbs MAGGI Fish Sauce
juice of 1 lime
1 tsp brown sugar
1 tsp sesame oil
500g beef strips
olive or canola oil spray
1 onion, halved and sliced

2 tsp minced garlic
1-2 tsp minced chilli
1 red capsicum, deseeded and
    finely sliced
1 bunch choy sum, shredded
100g bean sprouts
230g can bamboo shoots,
    rinsed and drained
1/4 cup roughly chopped fresh mint

Cook rice according to packet instructions. Combine oyster and fish sauces, lime juice and sugar in a small jug, set aside. Heat sesame oil in a non-stick wok or frypan over medium-high heat and stirfry beef in batches until browned. Remove and set aside. Spray wok/pan with oil, add onion, garlic, chilli and capsicum and stirfry until onion is soft. Add choy sum, bean sprouts and bamboo shoots and mix to combine. Return beef to pan, add sauce mixture and stir until heated through. Remove from heat and scatter with mint. Serve with rice.

Analysis	High Fuel	Low Fuel
	4	6
energy (kj)	2489	1405
● protein (g)	37	24
● fat (g)	8	5
● CHO (g)	90	46
● calcium, iron, vitamin C		

chicken & vegetable rice paper rolls Makes 12

dipping sauce:
1 tbs seasoned rice vinegar
juice of 1 lime
1 tbs caster sugar
1/4 cup MAGGI Fish Sauce
1-2 tsp minced chilli

rolls:
170g MAGGI 99% Fat Free
    2 Minute Noodles
200g asparagus, cut into 2cm lengths
    and blanched

12 x 20cm round rice paper sheets
100g enoki mushrooms
1 Lebanese cucumber, finely sliced
1 small carrot, peeled and grated
1 small red capsicum, deseeded
    and finely sliced
100g red cabbage, finely shredded
50g bamboo shoots, rinsed
    and drained
300g cooked chicken, shredded
1/2 cup fresh mint leaves
2 tbs chopped fresh chives

To make the dipping sauce, combine all the ingredients in a small jug or dish and set aside. Cook the noodles in boiling water for 2 minutes, until soft (do not add seasoning). Drain and then roughly chop. Heat asparagus in microwave on HIGH for 2 minutes or until just tender. Fill a large round dish with warm water. Place a sheet of rice paper in the water for about 2 minutes or until it softens. Gently remove from water and place on a clean tea towel. Place a small amount of noodles, asparagus, mushrooms, cucumber, carrot, capsicum, cabbage, bamboo shoots, chicken, mint and chives in the centre of the rice paper. Fold the bottom half of the rice paper over the filling and then fold in the sides and roll over to enclose the filling completely. Repeat with the remaining sheets of rice paper. Serve the rolls with the dipping sauce.
Note: This dish is a starter and should be combined with a meal.

Analysis	Per roll
energy (kj)	662
protein (g)	10
● fat (g)	5
CHO (g)	18

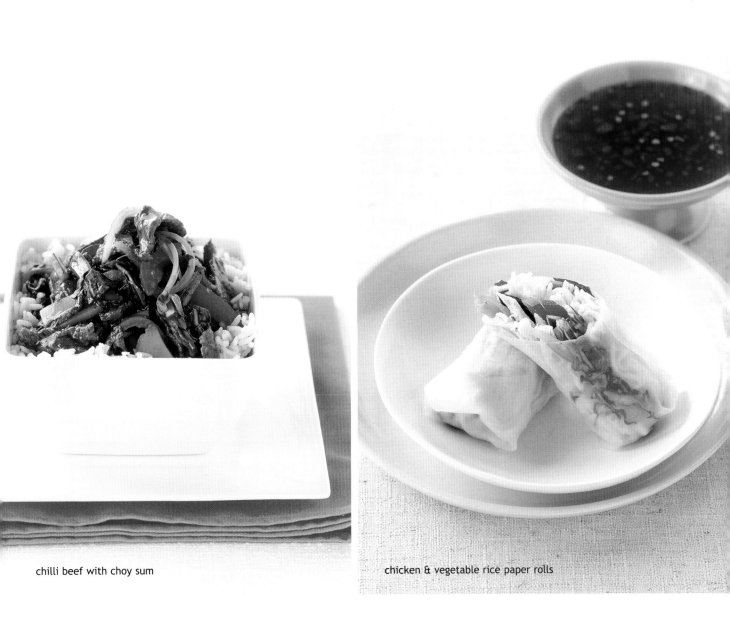

chilli beef with choy sum

chicken & vegetable rice paper rolls

"Knowing what to expect allowed us to plan for the nutritional needs of players during our tour to India. We took a range of safe snacks for times when the meals provided weren't up to scratch."

— AIS men's cricket team

indian beef curry Serves 4-6 ✳

2 cups rice	400g can crushed tomatoes
olive or canola oil spray	1 cup MAGGI Real Beef Stock
1 onion, chopped	1 zucchini, sliced
1 tsp ground coriander	1 cup sweet potato, diced
2 tsp ground cumin	150g green beans, cut into
2 tsp ground turmeric	4cm lengths
1 tsp minced garlic	2 tbs chopped fresh coriander
500g lean beef, cut into cubes	(optional)

Cook rice according to packet instructions. Spray a non-stick saucepan with oil and cook the onion, spices and garlic over medium heat for 2-3 minutes or until onion is golden. Add the beef and cook for 3-5 minutes or until brown. Add tomatoes and stock, reduce heat to low and simmer for 10 minutes. Add zucchini and sweet potato and simmer for a further 15-20 minutes or until tender. Add beans for the last 5 minutes of cooking. Sprinkle with coriander, if desired, and serve with rice.

Analysis	High Fuel 4	Low Fuel 6
energy (kj)	2599	1733
● protein (g)	42	28
● fat (g)	8	6
● CHO (g)	91	61
● iron, vitamin C		

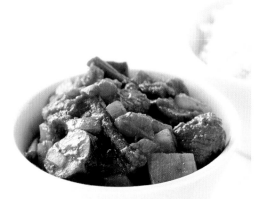

indian beef curry

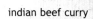

creating indian curries

▶ If you want a tangy flavour, add yogurt at the end of the cooking process.

▶ Evaporated milk and coconut essence make a great low-fat alternative to coconut milk or cream.

▶ Indian curries are often more delicious when eaten the next day. Store in an airtight container in the refrigerator and reheat.

thai chicken soup Serves 4-6 ✳

3/4 cup jasmine rice	4 kaffir lime leaves, finely shredded
olive or canola oil spray	1 tsp minced ginger
1 tsp green curry paste	500g chicken breast fillets,
1 litre MAGGI Real Chicken Stock	cut into thin strips
200ml CARNATION Light & Creamy	200g green beans, cut into
Evaporated Milk	3cm lengths
1 tsp coconut essence	1 red capsicum, deseeded and
1-2 red chillies, deseeded and	cut into thin strips
finely chopped	2 tsp honey
2 stems lemongrass, outer leaves	4 large or 6 small bread rolls
removed, finely chopped	

Cook rice according to packet instructions. Spray a non-stick saucepan with oil and cook curry paste over medium heat for 3 minutes, stirring occasionally. Add the stock, milk, coconut essence, chillies, lemongrass, lime leaves and ginger. Bring to the boil, then reduce heat to low, add chicken and simmer for a further 5-10 minutes or until chicken is cooked through. Add beans, capsicum, rice and honey and simmer for a further 5 minutes or until vegetables are tender. Serve with bread rolls, if desired.

Analysis	High Fuel 4	Low Fuel 6
energy (kj)	2572	1478
● protein (g)	45	28
● fat (g)	13	8
● CHO (g)	78	41
● calcium, iron, vitamin C		

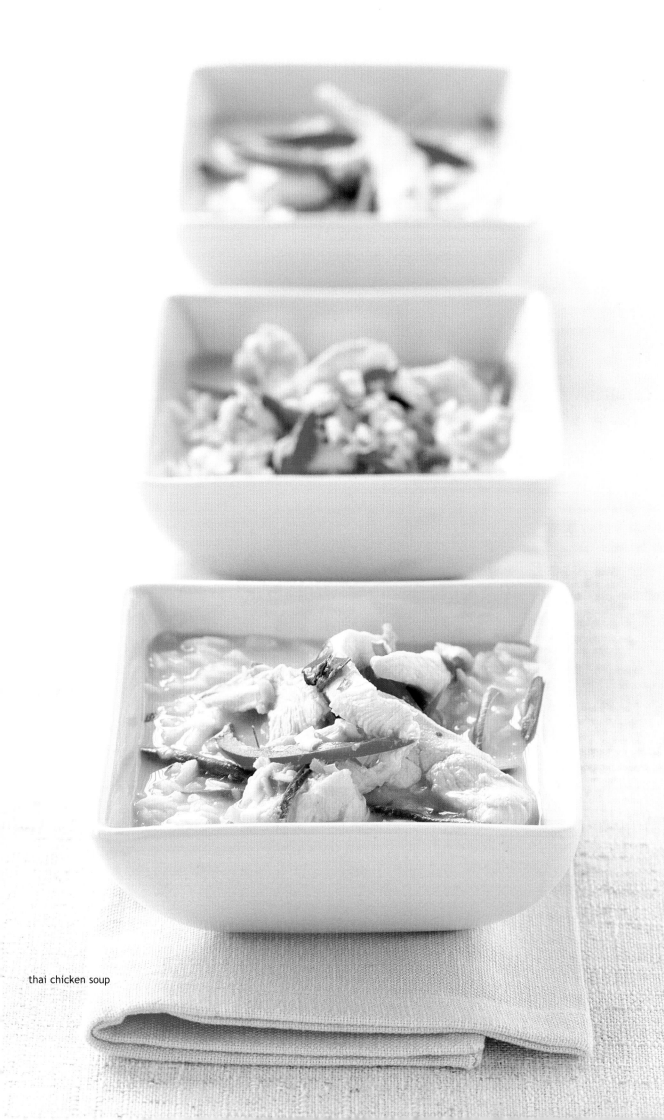

thai chicken soup

pork in black bean sauce Serves 4-6 ✳

2 cups rice
olive or canola oil spray
1 onion, cut into wedges
1 each small red and green capsicum,
    deseeded and sliced
1 large carrot, peeled and
    cut into thin strips

1 tsp minced garlic
500g pork fillets, sliced
1/4 cup black bean sauce
1 tsp MAGGI Sweet Chilli Sauce

Cook rice according to packet instructions. Spray a non-stick frypan with oil and cook onion, capsicums and carrot over medium heat for 2 minutes or until onion softens slightly. Transfer to a bowl. Add garlic and pork to pan and cook for 2 minutes or until browned. Return vegetables to pan, add sauces and cook for a further 2-3 minutes or until heated through. Serve with rice.

Analysis	High Fuel	Low Fuel
	4	6
energy (kj)	2372	1581
● protein (g)	35	24
● fat (g)	7	4
● CHO (g)	90	60
● calcium, iron, vitamin C		

tofu kebabs Serves 4-6

**You will need 12 bamboo skewers,
    soaked in water**
500g packet firm tofu, thickly sliced
    and cut into triangles
1/4 cup soy sauce
1 tsp minced garlic
11/2 tbs honey

2 cups rice
500g cherry tomatoes
2 zucchini, cut into four lengthways
    and thickly sliced
2 red onions, cut into wedges
green salad, to serve (optional)

Place tofu in a non-metallic container. Combine soy sauce, garlic and honey in a small bowl, then pour over tofu. Cover and refrigerate for 30 minutes to marinate. Meanwhile, cook rice according to packet instructions. Thread tomatoes, zucchini, onions and tofu alternately onto skewers (2 pieces of each per skewer). Preheat barbecue grill plate to medium-high heat. Cook, turning occasionally, for 5 minutes or until lightly charred. Serve with rice and a salad, if desired.

Analysis	High Fuel	Low Fuel
	4	6
energy (kj)	2439	1626
protein (g)	24	16
● fat (g)	9	6
● CHO (g)	97	65
● calcium, iron		

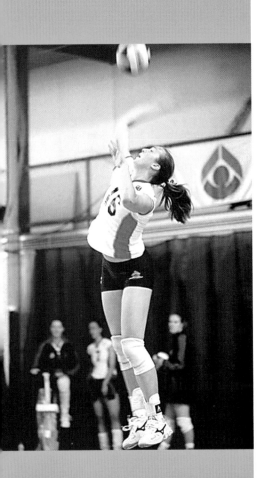

eileen romanowski — volleyball player

**Excerpt from *Ballad of Than Long*
by Eileen Romanowski**

Being experienced travellers, the girls
knew well,
Of cultures and their ways.
But nothing prepared them for
some things
That Vietnam portrays.

Water unguarded on the bench,
Was thrown to please the crowd,
But when Flo went for more supplies,
"NO NO!" That was not allowed.

Rations were made in the dining room,
One drink with every meal,
But when Lou brought her own
one day,
It became a big ordeal.

The meals were packed with spices,
Even chicken combs were served,
The girls watched mice happily
run past,
And ate their feed unnerved.

It was Flo who braved the water first,
The one without a seal.
It's a mistake she'd never make again,
'Cause of how it made her feel.

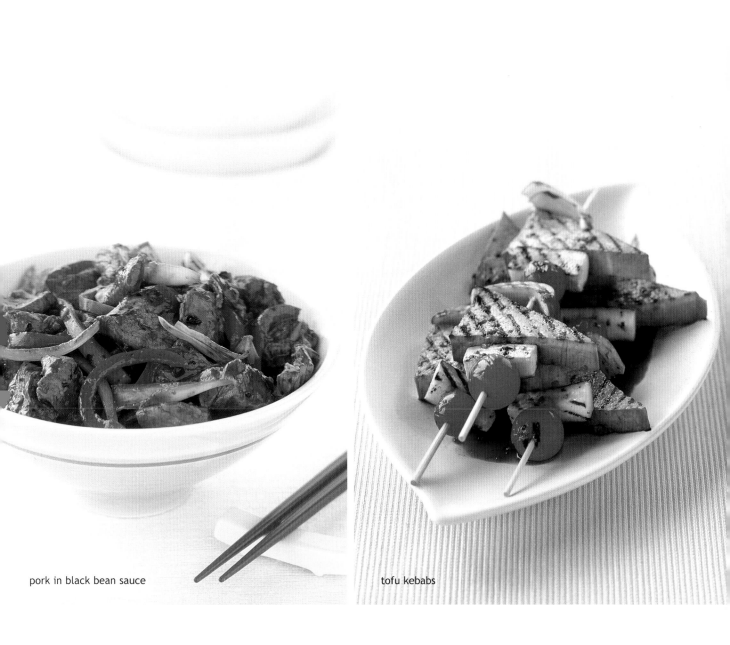

pork in black bean sauce

tofu kebabs

"Sweets in Japan can be misleading. What looked like pastry with chocolate spread in the middle turned out to be some kind of fishy, brown spread — sweet pastry and pureed fish!"
— AIS softball team

lamb biryani Serves 4-6 ✳

olive or canola oil spray
1 onion, chopped
2 tsp minced garlic
1 tbs minced ginger
2 tbs Indian curry paste (such as
  Madras or Tikka)
1 tsp ground cumin
1 tsp ground cinnamon
1 tsp ground turmeric
2 tsp ground coriander
500g lean lamb, cubed

1-1¹/₂ cups basmati rice
1 litre MAGGI Real Chicken Stock
1 cup frozen peas
200g cauliflower florets
¹/₄ cup diced dried apricots
200g PETERS FARM Natural
  No Fat Set Yogurt
2 tbs chopped fresh mint
2 tomatoes, chopped
2 tbs chopped fresh coriander

Preheat oven to 180°C (350°F). Spray a large casserole dish with oil and cook onion and garlic over medium heat until soft. Add ginger, curry paste, cumin, cinnamon, turmeric and ground coriander and cook, stirring, for 1 minute. Add ¹/₃ cup water, if necessary, to prevent sticking. Add lamb and cook for 3-5 minutes or until browned. Stir in rice and cook for 1 minute. Add stock, peas, cauliflower and apricots and bring to a simmer.

Analysis	High Fuel	Low Fuel
	4	6
energy (kj)	2679	1533
protein (g)	43	28
fat (g)	15	10
CHO (g)	78	39
calcium, iron, vitamin C		

Cover and then bake in oven for 25-30 minutes or until stock is absorbed and rice is cooked. Remove from oven and allow to rest for 5 minutes. Combine yogurt and mint. Combine tomatoes and coriander in a separate bowl. Serve biryani with yogurt mixture and tomato mixture.

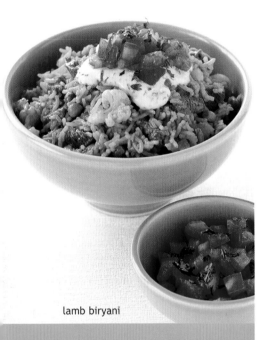

lamb biryani

the best biryani

▶ Biryani is used as a festive dish in India, to celebrate weddings and special events. It is one of the only Indian dishes that is served alone.

▶ Basmati rice is ideal for rice dishes that are cooked in the oven — this long-grain rice is low in starch, which means it won't stick to the other ingredients.

teriyaki chicken Serves 4-6 ✳

1¹/₂-2 cups sushi rice
  or soba noodles
500g chicken breast fillets, sliced
¹/₃ cup soy sauce
3 tbs mirin (sweet Japanese rice wine)
2 tbs caster sugar

2 cups MAGGI Real Chicken Stock
4 green shallots, diagonally sliced
300g broccoli florets
200g snow peas
1 red capsicum, deseeded and sliced
1 tbs cornflour

Cook rice or noodles according to packet instructions. Combine chicken, soy sauce, mirin and sugar in a non-metallic bowl and refrigerate for 30 minutes to marinate. Bring chicken mixture and stock to the boil in a saucepan, then reduce heat to low and simmer for 5 minutes. Add vegetables and simmer for 3 minutes, then cover and cook for a further 5 minutes. Mix cornflour with 1 tablespoon water and add to pan. Stir until sauce boils and thickens. Serve with rice or noodles.

Analysis	High Fuel	Low Fuel
	4	6
energy (kj)	2720	1561
protein (g)	42	27
fat (g)	8	6
CHO (g)	98	52
iron, vitamin C		

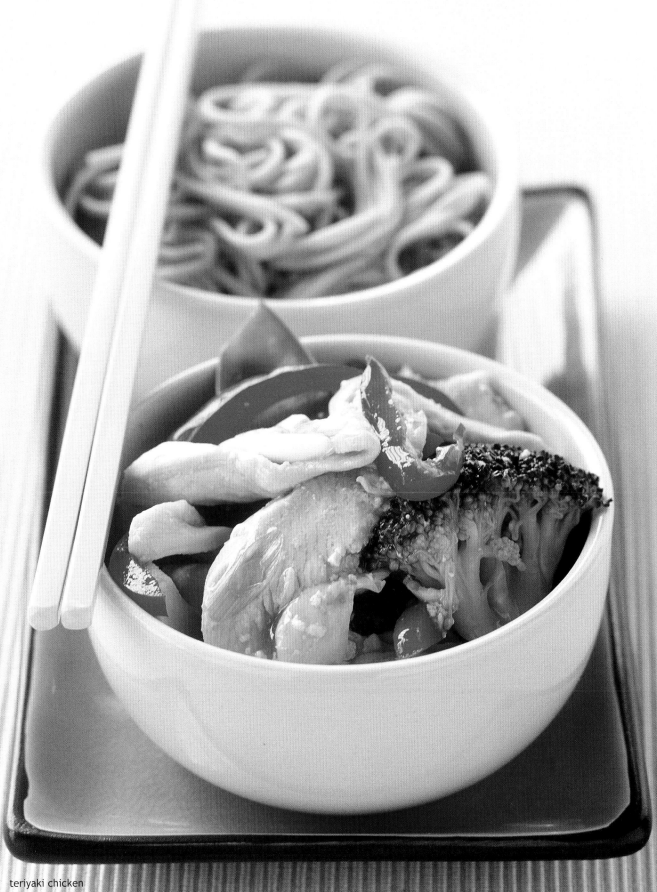

teriyaki chicken

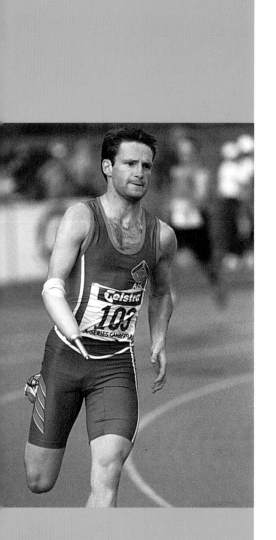

heath francis — paralympic 400m runner

"When I was overseas for competition, I went to a local food outlet and bought a chicken roll for lunch. The resulting food poisoning taught me to be very careful when buying food from outlets in areas where the risk of food contamination is high... choose carefully."

combination chow mein Serves 4-6 *

2 cups rice
olive or canola oil spray
150g green prawns, peeled and
  deveined with tails left intact
1¹/2 tsp minced garlic
200g beef, sliced
200g chicken breast fillet, sliced
1 cup broccoli florets
1 carrot, peeled and thinly sliced
6 button mushrooms, thinly sliced

¹/4 cup canned bamboo shoots,
  rinsed and drained
¹/2 cup snow peas, halved
1 small onion, thinly sliced
1 cup sliced cabbage
1 tbs MAGGI Fish Sauce
2 tbs MAGGI Oyster Sauce
2¹/2 tsp caster sugar
¹/4 tsp freshly ground black pepper

Cook rice according to packet instructions. Spray a non-stick wok or frypan with oil and stirfry prawns over high heat for 3 minutes or until opaque. Remove and set aside. Add garlic, beef and chicken and stirfry for 5 minutes or until cooked through. Add vegetables,

Analysis	High Fuel	Low Fuel
	4	6
energy (kj)	2417	1611
● protein (g)	40	26
● fat (g)	6	4
● CHO (g)	90	60
● iron, vitamin C		

sauces, sugar and pepper and stirfry for 2-3 minutes or until vegetables are just tender. Add prawns and stirfry until heated through. Serve with rice.
Tip: Use MAGGI Mince Chow Mein Recipe Mix as a short cut. Rice can be substituted with MAGGI 99% Fat Free 2 Minute Noodles.

asian pork salad in lettuce cups Serves 4-6 *

¹/2 cup rice
500g lean pork mince
¹/2 cup MAGGI Real Chicken Stock
230g can water chestnuts,
  drained and chopped
3 green shallots, chopped
2 tbs chopped fresh coriander
2 tbs chopped fresh mint

1 carrot, peeled and grated
1 cucumber, diced
3 tbs MAGGI Fish Sauce
2 tbs lime juice
1 tbs brown sugar
100g bean sprouts
1 iceberg lettuce, leaves separated
4 large or 6 small bread rolls

Cook rice according to packet instructions. Cook pork and stock in a non-stick frypan over medium heat for 10 minutes or until pork is tender. Remove from heat. Add rice,

Analysis	High Fuel	Low Fuel
	4	6
energy (kj)	2358	1580
● protein (g)	38	25
● fat (g)	13	9
● CHO (g)	70	46
● iron		

water chestnuts, green shallots, coriander, mint, carrot and cucumber and mix to combine. Whisk together fish sauce, lime juice and brown sugar and pour over pork mixture. Refrigerate for 1 hour or until chilled. Fold through bean sprouts and serve in lettuce leaves. Serve with bread rolls.

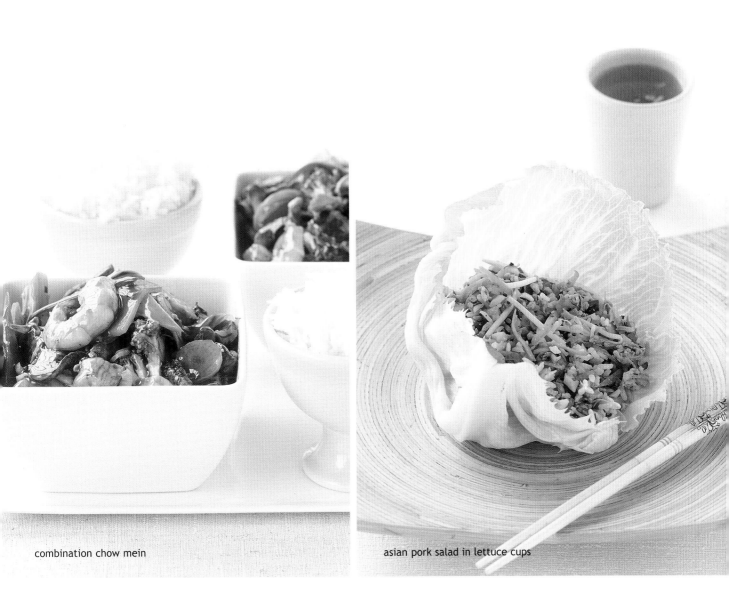

combination chow mein

asian pork salad in lettuce cups

"On our recent tour of Japan we were taken to a Japanese restaurant where we had to sit on the floor for a traditional meal. The funny thing was that they served us a Korean barbecue."
— deb cook, AIS women's basketball assistant coach

steamed pears Serves 4

4 pears (such as beurre bosc), peeled
4 tbs honey
pinch ground cinnamon

pinch ground nutmeg
400g NESTLÉ All Natural 99% Fat Free
   Vanilla Yogurt

Analysis	4 serves
energy (kj)	1109
protein (g)	6
fat (g)	<1
CHO (g)	58
calcium	

Cut tops off pears (these will become lids) and core. Stand pears upright in a bamboo steamer or steamer insert. Fill each pear with 1 tablespoon honey and sprinkle with cinnamon and nutmeg. Place top portion back on top of each pear. Cover, and place steamer over a saucepan of simmering water. Steam pears for 15-20 minutes or until soft. Serve with yogurt.

mango pudding Serves 4-6

You will need 4-6 jelly moulds or
  1-cup serving dishes
6 tsp gelatine powder
3/4 cup caster sugar
3 cups pureed mango
  (fresh or canned)

1 cup CARNATION Light & Creamy
  Evaporated Milk
8 ice cubes
juice and zest of 2 limes, to serve
fresh mango (or your choice of fruit),
  chopped, to garnish (optional)

Heat 1 cup water in a small saucepan over low heat. Add gelatine and sugar and stir until gelatine dissolves and mixture is smooth. Set aside to cool. In a large bowl, combine

Analysis	High Fuel	Low Fuel
	4	6
energy (kj)	1133	756
protein (g)	11	7
fat (g)	<1	<1
CHO (g)	56	37
calcium, vitamin C		

mango puree, milk and ice cubes. Pour gelatine mixture into mango mixture and stir until ice cubes melt. Pour mixture into 6 jelly moulds or dishes and refrigerate for at least 3 hours or until set. To serve, squeeze a little lime juice over puddings and garnish with mango/fruit pieces and lime zest.

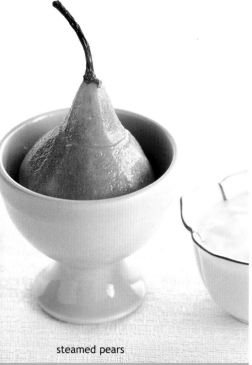

steamed pears

cooking with pears

▶ In addition to steaming, pears can also be poached, grilled, baked, sauteed, microwaved or barbecued. Adding a little honey or sugar to them when cooking will enhance their flavour.

▶ Pears can be substituted for apples in most recipes.

▶ If you have peeled or cut pears, but are not using them straight away, brush with a little lemon juice to prevent them discolouring.

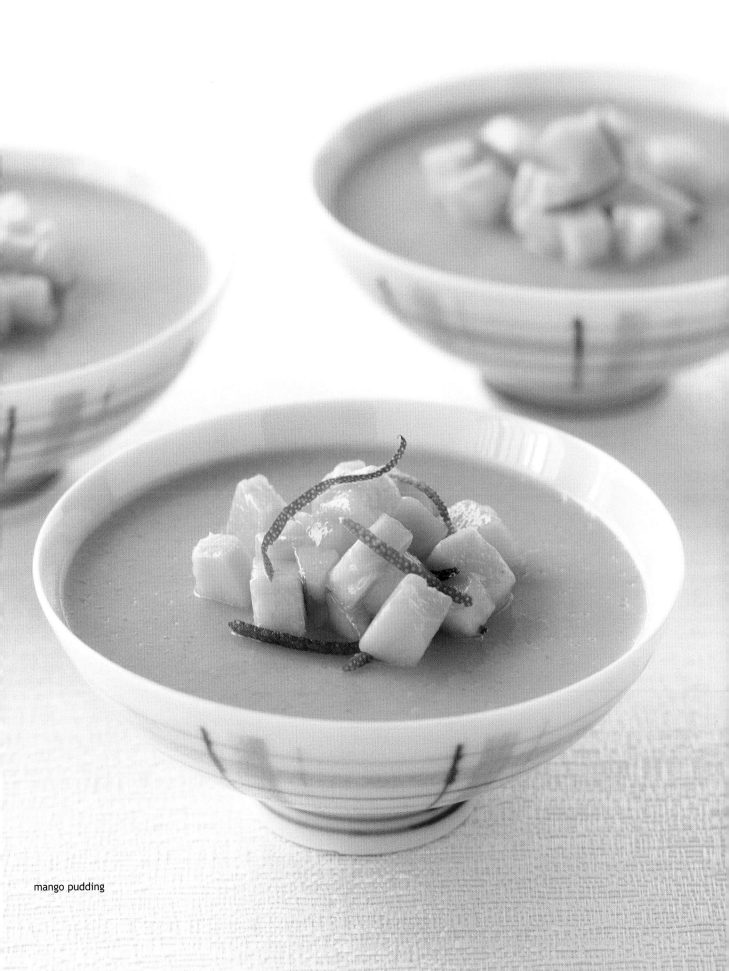

mango pudding

middle east

Dining is a true family affair in the Middle East — long tables are laden with a sumptuous selection of meat and vegetable dishes and meals seem to last for hours. Chicken and lamb kebabs, stews and pides are accompanied by a variety of salads, breads and dips, with fragrant spices and lively conversation adding a distinct flavour.

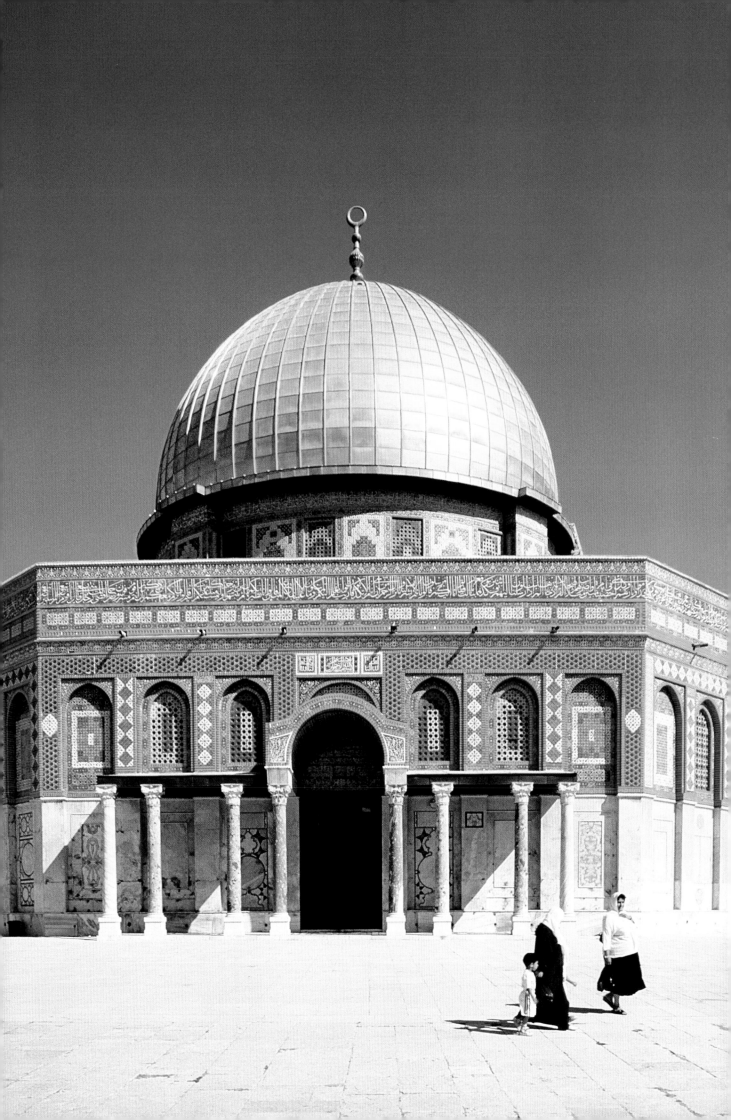

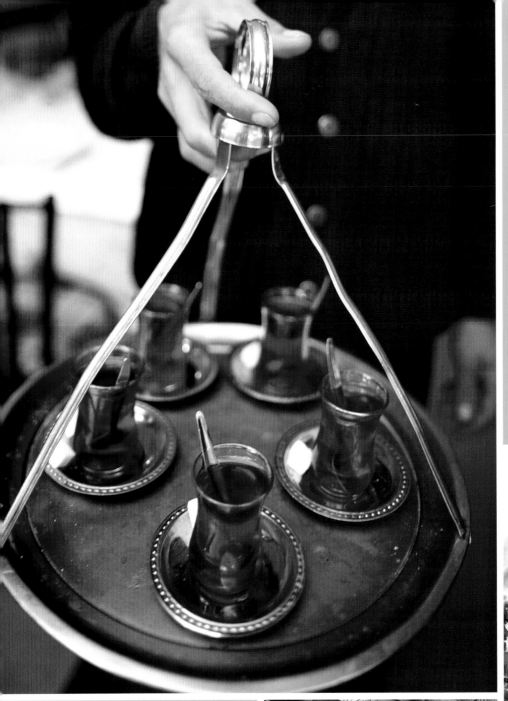

food availability

Both international and traditional restaurants are plentiful throughout Middle Eastern cities and towns. Grilled lamb and chicken kebabs, mezze, rice dishes, vegetables and salads are recommended traditional choices. Bread always accompanies meals. Fresh produce can be purchased throughout the Middle East in souqs (markets) (shuks in Israel) or supermarkets. Bread, fresh fruit, vegetables and sweet pastries are readily available. It is important to check for good refrigeration before purchasing meats – slabs of meat often sit in markets for hours, uncovered and unrefrigerated. Sports drinks, gels, powders and bars are difficult to find in the Middle East. It is advisable to take a supply from home.

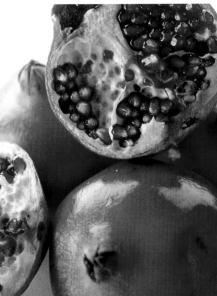

about the culture

Fragrant spices, such as turmeric, cumin, cloves and cinnamon feature strongly in Middle Eastern cuisine. Lamb, chicken, rice, goat's milk, dates, nuts, fresh fruit, yogurt and tomatoes are also common ingredients. Breakfast usually consists of bread eaten with dips, cheese, honey, jam, vegetables and cheese. Lunch is often the main meal of the day and may be consumed as late as 2-3pm. The meal will often begin with an entrée called mezze – a selection of foods in small dishes, such as dips and dolmas (stuffed grape leaves). The main course can include felafels (deep-fried chickpea balls), kebabs of grilled lamb or chicken, lamb stew, rice dishes, fruits and nuts. Dessert is usually only eaten when entertaining, and nut-filled desserts, such as baklavá or almond cookies, rice pudding flavoured with rosewater and sweet dairy snacks are the most popular choices. The evening meal is usually lighter than lunch but consists of similar dishes.

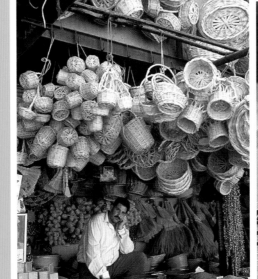

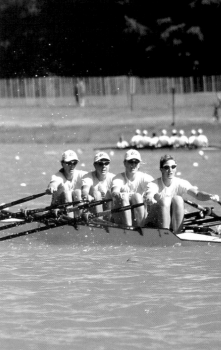

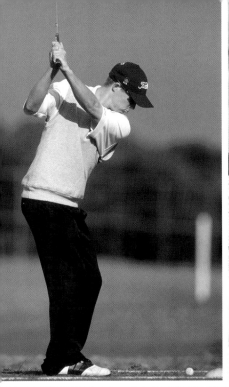

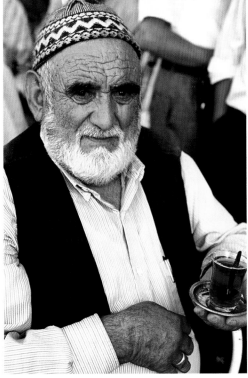

useful tips

▶ The risk of food poisoning from
  contaminated foods and water is high.
  Care is required at all times, whether
  eating in restaurants or self-catering

▶ During Ramadan, the annual month-long
  fast during which Muslims abstain from
  food and drink from dawn till dusk, most
  restaurants close until sundown. Shops
  may be open for a few hours during the
  morning and a short time after the
  breaking of the fast

▶ Take your own food and fluid supplies
  to training and competition venues as
  they usually won't have kiosks that sell
  your regular snack choices

▶ Meals are served communally, from the
  same dish and eaten with the thumb
  and first two fingers of the right hand.

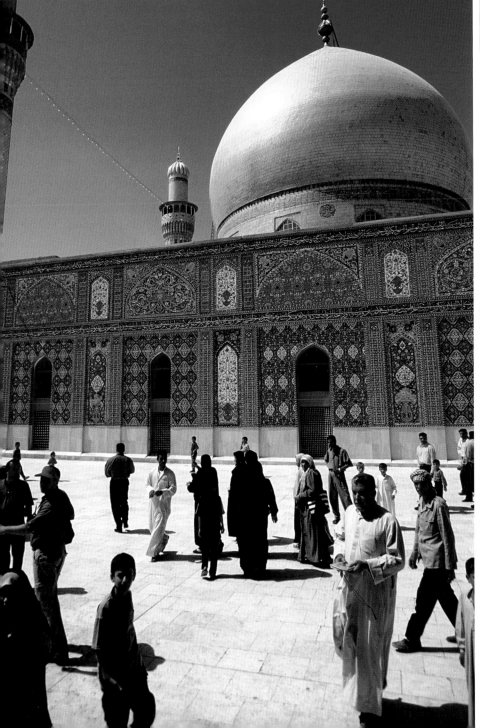

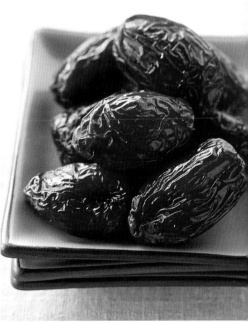

main nutrient sources

carbohydrate

Rice, bread and legumes, such as black
beans, chickpeas, lentils, navy beans and
red beans. Fresh fruit and vegetables are
also widely available

protein

Lamb and poultry are popular. Pork is rare,
as both Jewish and Muslim faiths forbid
the eating of this meat. Most dairy
products are eaten in fermented forms,
such as yogurt. Feta is the most
commonly used cheese

fat

Olive oil is used liberally in Middle
Eastern cuisine.

turkish pide pizza

Makes 2 pizzas (serves 4-6) ✳

2¹/2 cups plain flour
7g sachet dried yeast
1 tsp salt
1 tbs olive oil, plus extra
   to grease

Combine flour, yeast and salt in a bowl. Make a well in the centre and mix in oil and 250-300ml lukewarm water until a soft dough forms. Turn dough out onto a lightly floured surface and knead for 3 minutes or until almost smooth. Place dough in a clean, lightly greased bowl. Cover with plastic wrap and leave in a warm place for about 1 hour or until doubled in size. Preheat oven to 200°C (400°F). Punch dough down with your fist and knead for 30 seconds or until dough returns to its original size. Cut dough in half and roll into 2 oval shapes, about 1cm thick. Place dough on a baking tray lined with non-stick paper. Place filling (see recipes on this page) in the centre and fold in sides to partially enclose filling. Squeeze dough together at each end. Lightly brush with olive oil or water. Bake for about 20 minutes or until crisp and golden.

fillings:

spinach, feta & potato   For 2 pizzas (serves 4-6)

1 large potato, cut into small cubes
250g frozen spinach, defrosted and
   excess water squeezed out

200g low-fat feta, crumbled
2 eggs, lightly whisked

Analysis	High Fuel	Low Fuel
	4	6
energy (kj)	2390	1593
protein (g)	29	20
fat (g)	17	12
CHO (g)	70	47
calcium		

Heat potato in microwave on HIGH for 3-5 minutes or until par-cooked. Combine with remaining ingredients.

chicken, cheese & tomato   For 2 pizzas (serves 4-6)

100g low-fat hummus
400g cooked chicken breast fillets,
   shredded
1/4 cup grated low-fat cheese

2 tomatoes, diced
2 tbs chopped fresh flat-leaf parsley,
   to garnish

Analysis	High Fuel	Low Fuel
	4	6
energy (kj)	2406	1604
protein (g)	38	26
fat (g)	15	10
CHO (g)	68	45

Spread dough with hummus, then top with chicken, cheese and tomatoes. When pizzas are cooked, sprinkle with parsley.

lamb   For 2 pizzas (serves 4-6)

olive or canola oil spray
1 small onion, finely chopped
1 tsp minced garlic
500g minced trim lamb
1/2 tsp ground cinnamon
1 tsp mixed spice

1 tbs lemon juice
2 tomatoes, diced
1/3 cup PETERS FARM Natural
   No Fat Set Yogurt, to garnish
2 tbs chopped fresh mint,
   to garnish

Analysis	High Fuel	Low Fuel
	4	6
energy (kj)	2230	1486
protein (g)	32	22
fat (g)	13	9
CHO (g)	67	45
iron		

Spray a non-stick frypan with oil and cook onion and garlic over medium heat until soft. Add mince, spices and lemon juice and cook until brown. Remove from heat and stir tomatoes through. When pizzas are cooked, drizzle with yogurt and sprinkle with mint.

tomato, mushroom & capsicum   For 2 pizzas (serves 4-6)

1/2 cup tahini
1 tsp minced garlic
100g mushrooms
1/2 cup grated low-fat cheese

2 tomatoes, diced
1 small green capsicum, deseeded
   and diced
2 tbs chopped fresh chives, to garnish

Analysis	High Fuel	Low Fuel
	4	6
energy (kj)	2196	1464
protein (g)	19	13
fat (g)	19	13
CHO (g)	66	44

Combine tahini and garlic and spread over dough. Top with mushrooms, cheese, tomatoes and capsicum. When pizzas are cooked, sprinkle with chives.

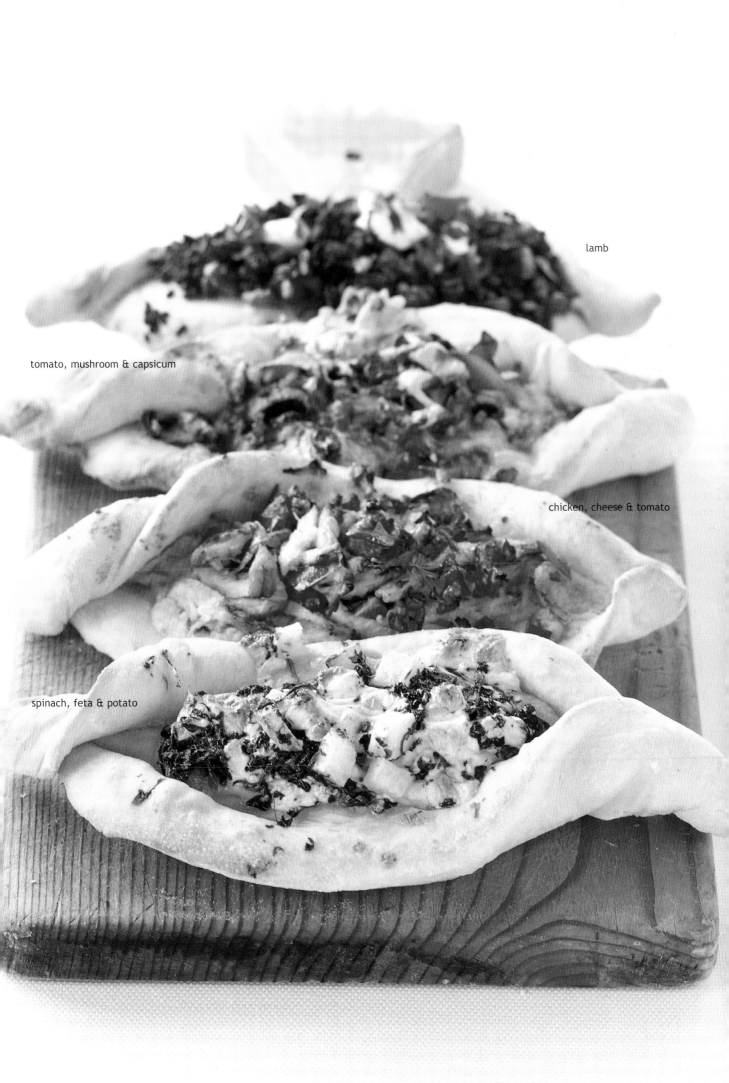

lamb

tomato, mushroom & capsicum

chicken, cheese & tomato

spinach, feta & potato

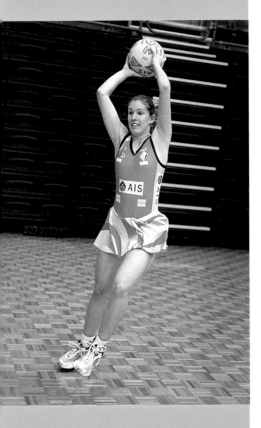

kirby mutton — netball player

"When travelling last year, we had stopovers in unfamiliar countries. We were prepared for the food at our final destination, but hadn't considered the stopovers. The meals were unrecognisable. Our dietitian had provided 'travel packs' consisting of snacks and drinks for the flight which helped. Next time, we will plan further and make sure we're prepared for the food everywhere we go."

chicken tagine with couscous Serves 4-6

olive or canola oil spray
2 onions, halved and sliced
2 tsp minced garlic
3 baby eggplants, diced
2 tsp each ground cumin and coriander
1 tsp each ground turmeric and cinnamon
500g chicken breast fillets,
    cut into chunks
400g can chopped tomatoes
grated rind and juice of 1 lemon
1¹/2 cups MAGGI Real Chicken Stock

¹/4 cup pitted black olives, halved
2 small zucchini, chopped
¹/2 cup dried apricots, diced
1 tbs chopped fresh coriander,
    to garnish (optional)

couscous:
1¹/2-2 cups couscous
¹/2 cup MAGGI Real Chicken Stock
1 tbs chopped fresh coriander
    (optional)

Spray a non-stick saucepan with oil and cook onions, garlic and eggplants over medium heat until soft. Add cumin, coriander, turmeric and cinnamon and cook for 1 minute. Add chicken and cook until browned. Add tomatoes, lemon rind and juice, stock, olives, zucchini and apricots and simmer for 20-30 minutes. Meanwhile, to make couscous, cover couscous with stock and 1 cup boiling water. Set aside for 5 minutes or until liquid is absorbed. Fluff with a fork and stir fresh coriander through, if desired. Serve tagine over couscous. Garnish with fresh coriander, if desired.

Analysis	High Fuel 4	Low Fuel 6
energy (kj)	3010	1613
protein (g)	43	26
fat (g)	12	8
CHO (g)	105	50
iron, vitamin C		

kofta kebabs with tabouli Serves 4-6 ✳

350g trim lamb mince
¹/2 onion, grated
¹/2 tsp allspice
¹/4 tsp ground cinnamon
¹/2 cup cracked wheat (burghul)

tabouli:
¹/3 cup cracked wheat
4 cups chopped fresh flat-leaf parsley

1¹/4 cups chopped fresh mint
3 ripe tomatoes, diced
4 green shallots, sliced
juice of 2 lemons
canola or olive oil spray, to grease
250g hummus, to serve
6-12 small Lebanese breads, to serve

Combine lamb, onion and spices in a bowl. Rinse wheat under cold water and drain well. Add to meat mixture and mix thoroughly to combine. Shape mixture into 12 sausage shapes. Cover and refrigerate for 20 minutes. Meanwhile, to make tabouli, soak wheat in cold water for 10 minutes, then drain well to remove excess water. Combine with parsley, mint, tomatoes and green shallots. Pour lemon juice over salad, toss to combine. Preheat a lightly oiled barbecue flat plate to medium-high heat. Cook kebabs, turning occasionally, for 10 minutes or until cooked through. Serve with hummus and bread.

Analysis	High Fuel 4	Low Fuel 6
energy (kj)	2926	1414
protein (g)	40	22
fat (g)	11	7
CHO (g)	101	43
calcium, iron, vitamin C		

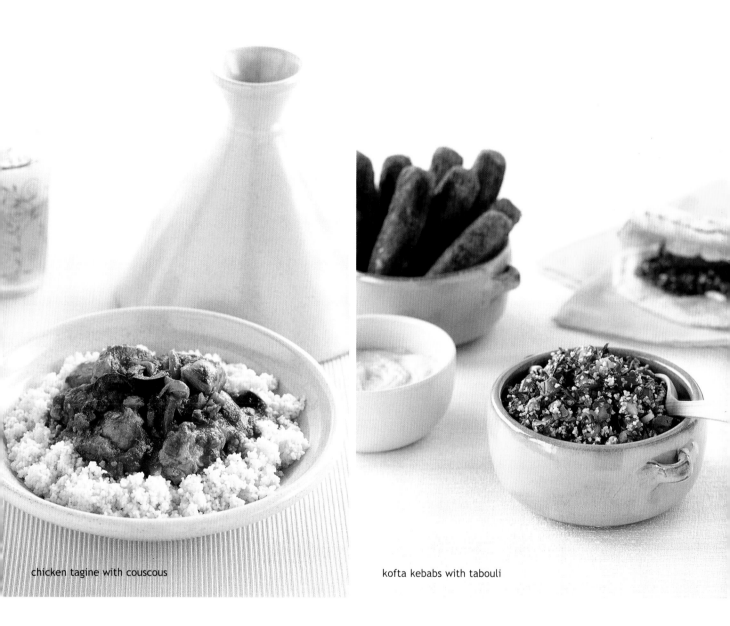

chicken tagine with couscous

kofta kebabs with tabouli

"Travelling overseas often requires great restraint. When staying in hotels with an array of different food choices at every meal, it takes self-discipline to choose foods that are in line with my usual eating patterns. I still want to perform at my best and don't want to be caught off guard by eating foods I am not familiar with. Another way I cope is to take breakfast cereal and snack foods with me to supplement the potentially unusual cuisine."

— craig stevens, swimmer

creamed rice with spiced apples Serves 4-6

1 cup arborio rice
1/2 cup caster sugar
3 cups CARNATION Light & Creamy
   Evaporated Milk
4 red apples, cored and cut into wedges

1 cinnamon stick
pinch saffron threads (optional)
1/4 cup brown sugar
1 cup apple juice

Place rice and 2 cups water in a saucepan, bring to the boil, without stirring, and cook over medium heat for 5 minutes or until most of water is absorbed. Add caster sugar and milk and bring to the boil. Reduce heat to low and simmer for 20 minutes, stirring occasionally to prevent sticking, until rice is soft. Meanwhile, place remaining ingredients in a saucepan and stir over low heat until brown sugar dissolves. Bring to the boil, reduce heat to low and simmer, covered, for 5-10 minutes or until apples are just soft. Remove cinnamon stick. Serve rice topped with apples and cooking liquid.

Analysis	High Fuel	Low Fuel
	4	6
energy (kj)	2392	1595
● protein (g)	19	13
● fat (g)	1	<1
● CHO (g)	122	81
● calcium		

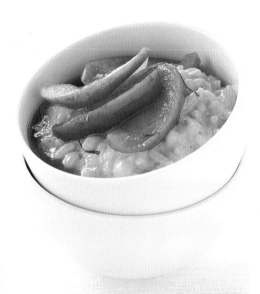

creamed rice with spiced apples

layered fruits with lemon pistachio syrup Serves 4-6

800g watermelon, peeled and sliced
2 mangoes, sliced
2 pears, sliced
3 kiwifruit, peeled and sliced
250g strawberries, hulled and sliced
150g fresh or frozen blueberries
1 vanilla bean, split and scraped,
   or 1 tsp vanilla essence

1/2 cup caster sugar
2 tsp lemon zest
1 tsp rosewater essence
50g pistachio kernels,
   roughly chopped
400g PETERS FARM Natural No Fat
   Set Yogurt, to serve (optional)

Layer fruits in a large serving bowl. Place vanilla bean/essence, sugar, lemon zest, rosewater essence and 1 1/2 cups water in a saucepan and bring to the boil. Reduce heat and simmer for 15 minutes or until slightly thickened. Allow to cool, strain. Pour syrup over fruits and sprinkle with pistachios. Serve with yogurt, if desired.

Analysis	High Fuel	Low Fuel
	4	6
energy (kj)	1915	1276
● protein (g)	13	8
● fat (g)	7	5
● CHO (g)	80	53
● calcium, vitamin C		

terrific toppings

▶ You can serve this creamy rice with lots of different toppings, depending on what is available to you.

▶ Fresh berries, such as raspberries, strawberries and/or blueberries, with a light drizzling of honey.

▶ Replace the apples in the recipe with pears.

▶ Fruit salad, such as bananas, peaches and kiwifruit, topped with passionfruit pulp and/or a little fresh orange juice.

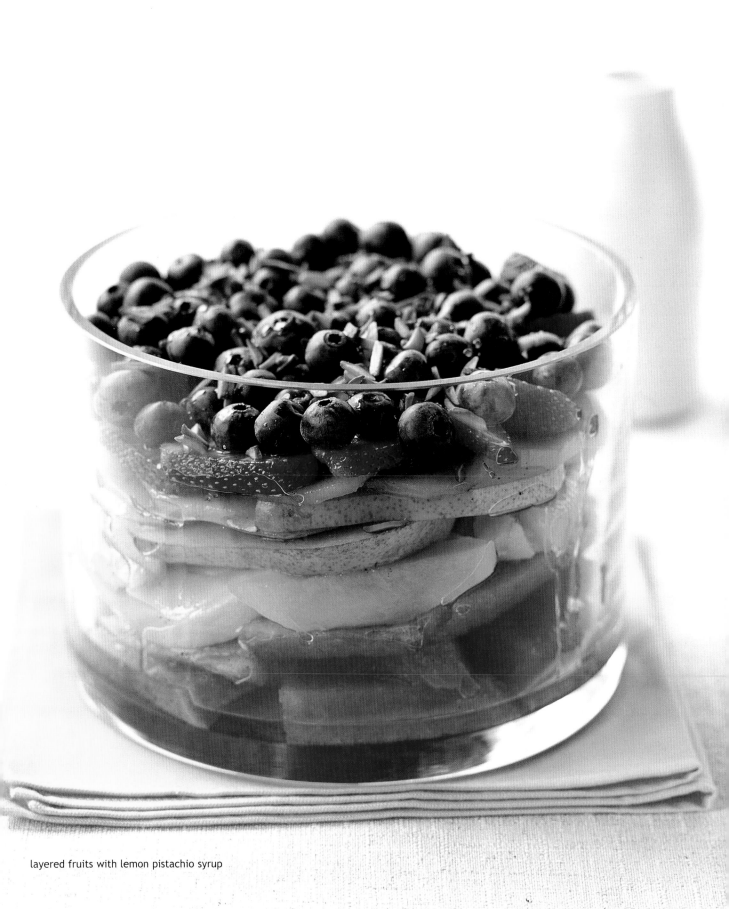

layered fruits with lemon pistachio syrup

how to stay on track

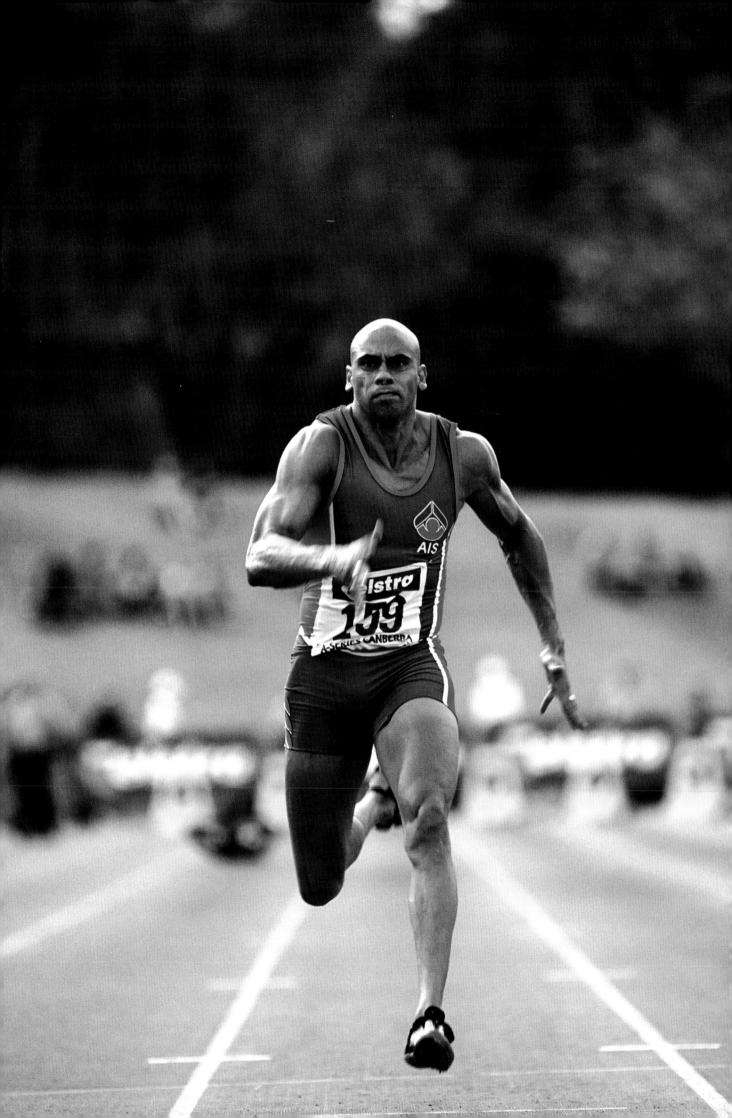

eating out

Relying on restaurants is an expensive option for travelling athletes, however, you may find yourself in a situation where you can cater for your own breakfasts and lunches and eat out in the evenings. Restaurants offer a variety of choices; the trick is to make sure you pick the right restaurant and the right menu item in order to stay on track with your nutrition goals.

plan ahead

- Where possible, restaurants should be investigated before leaving home. The meal options, cooking styles, opening hours and hygiene of the establishment should be considered. The Internet, travel agencies, competition organisers, embassies or other athletes who have previously travelled to the destination can be used to gain valuable information
- When travelling as a large group, it is useful to book restaurants ahead of time as many businesses are unable to cater for specific requests or large groups at short notice
- Discuss the proposed menu with restaurant staff in advance to minimise problems at meal time. This is particularly important when athletes have special dietary needs (e.g. vegetarian, food intolerances).

basic rules for eating out

- Make sure that your water glass is regularly topped up to help with hydration goals. When extra carbohydrate is needed, soft drinks or fruit juice may also be a good option
- When fuel needs are high, order a basket of plain bread to boost the carbohydrate in your meal
- Choose meals that focus on carbohydrate, such as rice or pasta. Opt for sauces without cream and with low levels of cheese and oil
- If you are having a main course based on meat, fish or poultry, choose a medium-sized portion and don't forget the fuel foods, such as a baked potato or a side dish of rice
- Order side serves of vegetables or salad if they don't come with the meal. Ask for black pepper, tomato sauce or salsa rather than buttery sauces, and lemon juice or balsamic vinegar rather than salad dressings. You can always order dressing on the side, and then you can add the desired amount to suit your needs
- Desserts are not mandatory – keep your overall nutrition goals in mind. Carbohydrate-rich desserts include rice pudding, bread and butter pudding, sorbet, fruit salad or fruit crumble and custard. If you're watching your total energy intake, finish with a fruit platter or a skim-milk hot chocolate.

mexican restaurants

- Always steer clear of high-fat fried options, such as corn chips
- Enchiladas and burritos are often a good choice, however check the fillings for high-fat ingredients, such as cheese and cream. Some enchiladas and burritos can be drowned in cheese and also cheese-filled
- Be mindful of sour cream and guacamole. Ask to have these on the side so you can adjust the amount to suit your needs
- Fajitas are generally a well-balanced option, especially when served with rice and frijole (refried beans).

italian restaurants

- Plain Italian bread is a great accompaniment to your meal. Be careful not to overindulge in flavoured breads, such as garlic, pesto, sun-dried tomato or herb if you need to keep your fat intake low
- Tomato-based pasta sauces, such as napolitana, marinara and bolognaise are all great options. Be wary of high-fat sauces based on pesto or cream, such as carbonara
- Pizzas can be a great option, especially when you choose your own toppings. If you're aiming to reduce the fat content in the meal, choose low-fat meats and a small amount of cheese
- Traditional menu items, such as fried calamari and veal parmagiana are high-fat options – steer clear of these if you are aiming to keep your fat intake down.

indian restaurants

▮ Add plain steamed rice to your plate to ensure your meal is based around carbohydrate

▮ Accompaniments, such as roti, paratha or chapatti (all varieties of flat bread) provide a fuel boost to a meal

▮ Many curry sauces can be high in fat. Control the fat content of your meal by serving a small amount of sauce with plenty of rice. Also order vegetable dishes.

asian restaurants

Authentic Vietnamese, Thai, Japanese and Korean restaurants offer a great range of nutritious choices for the athlete. Keep in mind that Chinese restaurants in Australia tend to offer more high-fat choices.

▮ Steamed rice or noodles should make up the bulk of your plate. Wheat noodles, such as Hokkien tend to be higher in carbohydrate than rice noodles

▮ Choose combination dishes that include a good variety of vegetables, otherwise order some separate steamed vegetables to balance your meal

▮ Avoid dishes that are deep-fried or battered

▮ Be wary of entrées, as many of these are deep-fried, such as spring rolls, dim sims, tempura and chicken wings. Sushi and rice paper rolls are good options.

cafés

▮ Sandwiches based on regular, Turkish and Italian breads are all good starting points to build a great meal

▮ Hamburgers can be an excellent choice. Make sure they are grilled and have plenty of added salad. Choose tomato sauce rather than mayonnaise or creamy dressings and avoid extras such as double meat, fried eggs, bacon or cheese

▮ Soup with bread is a good choice provided it does not contain a lot of cream

▮ Be careful with Caesar salads and quiche – these are often the highest fat choices

▮ Most cafés offer a selection of milks – always specify if you want full-cream, reduced-fat or skim

▮ Be careful with the selection of muffins, cakes, slices and pastries available at cafés. Most are high in fat and the serving size is usually very large.

takeaways

Takeaway food can be a cheap and convenient option while travelling. Takeaway outlets are often the only shops open, or the only place offering familiar and hygienically prepared food. Although many takeaway food choices are high in fat and low on fuel, there are some good choices available. Follow these tips:

▮ Look for chains or outlets that let you make your own order instead of those serving standard products. Salad bars are ideal, but avoid meal deals which, although cheap, see you eating extra fries or fatty desserts that you don't really need

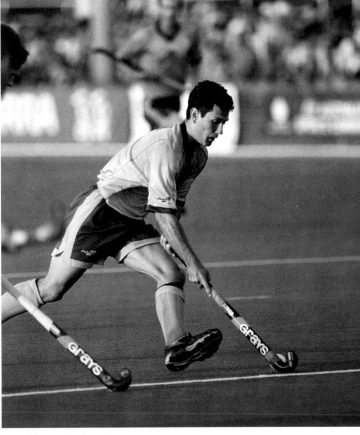

ben bishop – hockey player

▮ Make good use of the nutritional information that is provided at many franchises

▮ When ordering pizza, choose your own toppings. Include plenty of vegetables and go easy on processed meats and cheese

▮ Baked potatoes are an excellent takeaway choice. Avoid butter or sour cream toppings and select toppings such as tuna, baked beans, salsa or bolognaise sauce

▮ Kebabs or souvlaki are one of the better takeaway choices. Take care with some creamy dressings

▮ Fish and chips are a high-fat choice, however a fish burger made with grilled fish and plenty of salad can be a good option.

self-catering

Many small groups or individuals choose to stay in apartments and do their own cooking when away on trips. This can be an economical choice that also offers flexibility with meal times and food selections.

However, as with cooking at home, it can be hard to find the motivation and appetite to prepare a meal when you are exhausted from an event or training, and there are added problems with organising menus for limited stays. It is hard to coordinate dishes that can be made from a limited number of ingredients, and often you end up with leftovers or unused ingredients, or you may find your favourite dish doesn't taste the same without a pinch of something you don't have.

Quick and easy meals that require a minimum number of ingredients and equipment are essential, and the following menus are designed with this in mind. First, we have provided a full menu plan for a week (Seven-day Menu Plan), in which meal selections are balanced and coordinated to use up leftovers. The second menu plan (Quick & Easy Dinner Menu), caters for evening meals only and mixes and matches the recipes so that all ingredients are used. For both plans, we've included a shopping list of all the ingredients you will need.

notes on the shopping lists:

▶ If you need to save lots of time, contact the local supermarket at your destination and ask if they will collect and deliver your shopping needs. Fax your shopping list to them before you arrive and arrange for the items to be delivered shortly before or after your arrival

▶ Snack needs vary according to the individual, so you should add them to the list according to your requirements

▶ Take advantage of local or seasonal produce, such as fresh fruit and vegetables or bread and simply adjust the shopping list accordingly

▶ Under 'Miscellaneous' in the shopping list are many foods that are required in small amounts. The sauces, seasonings and herbs may be purchased with the other supplies, or you may like to take your own. These can be placed in small jars, plastic bags or tubes (such as clean film canisters) and then the whole lot packed into a larger airtight container. You can also leave some of the sauces out of the recipes, or substitute according to what's available.

seven-day menu plan

This menu plan will provide four athletes with three meals per day (breakfast, lunch and dinner) for a week. The recipes from *Survival Around the World* have page numbers listed for easy reference.

all you need to do is:

▶ Check that the recipe suggestions suit your needs and make alterations as necessary

▶ If possible, check the availability of cooking equipment in your apartment. You may need to adjust the recipes if important cooking equipment is missing. Alternatively, you can take a time-saving or versatile piece of cooking equipment with you

▶ Pack *Survival Around the World*

▶ Follow the shopping list and buy the ingredients.

equipment

▶ Stove top
▶ Oven
▶ Non-stick frying pan or wok
▶ Large saucepan
▶ Ovenproof dish or baking tray
▶ Microwave
▶ Microwave dishes
▶ Wooden spoon or large plastic spoons
▶ Selection of knives
▶ Chopping board.

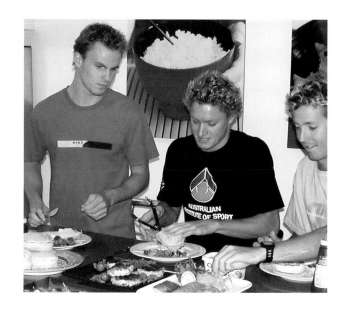

shopping list:

bread
- [ ] 5 loaves of bread
- [ ] 4 bagels
- [ ] 8 bread rolls
- [ ] 8 large burrito flour tortillas
- [ ] 1 packet pikelets
- [ ] 2 pizza bases

fruit & vegetables
- [ ] 8 large potatoes
- [ ] 5 large onions
- [ ] 500g mushrooms
- [ ] 20 large tomatoes
- [ ] 11 large carrots
- [ ] 8 Lebanese cucumbers
- [ ] 2 red capsicums
- [ ] 2 green capsicums
- [ ] 10 zucchini
- [ ] 2 leeks
- [ ] 6 green shallots
- [ ] 4 celery sticks
- [ ] 2 iceberg lettuces
- [ ] 500g mixed lettuce
- [ ] 200g rocket
- [ ] 1 bunch flat-leaf parsley
- [ ] 100g sun-dried tomatoes (no oil)
- [ ] 20 apples (at least 4 red)
- [ ] 14 bananas
- [ ] 2 punnets strawberries
- [ ] 2 kiwifruit
- [ ] 6 large nectarines
- [ ] 12 pears
- [ ] 2 lemons

dairy & refrigerated products
- [ ] 7 litres fruit juice (including apple)
- [ ] 5 litres reduced-fat or skim milk
- [ ] 200g ultra-light sour cream (10% fat)
- [ ] 2 x 1 litre NESTLÉ All Natural 99% Fat Free Vanilla Yogurt
- [ ] 3 x 1 litre NESTLÉ All Natural 99% Fat Free Fruit Yogurt
- [ ] 500g grated reduced-fat cheese
- [ ] 250g grated parmesan cheese
- [ ] 200g low-fat spreadable cream cheese
- [ ] 500g canola margarine

canned & packaged products
- [ ] 300g textured vegetable protein (TVP) mince
- [ ] 3 x 500g breakfast cereals (vary according to your preference)
- [ ] 2 x 450g cans baked beans
- [ ] 2 x 400g cans spaghetti
- [ ] 435g can refried beans
- [ ] 400g can creamed corn
- [ ] 300g can corn kernels
- [ ] 4 x 400g cans tomatoes
- [ ] 400g can beetroot

- [ ] 2 x 400g cans tuna in spring water/brine
- [ ] 12 x 400g cans fruit (vary according to your preference)
- [ ] 300g can pineapple rings in natural juice
- [ ] 375g spiral pasta
- [ ] 1kg long-grain rice
- [ ] 2kg arborio rice
- [ ] 600g chunky salsa
- [ ] 500g tomato paste
- [ ] 1 packet Anzac biscuits
- [ ] 1 packet pancake mix
- [ ] 4 x 375ml, 1 x 150ml CARNATION Light & Creamy Evaporated Milk
- [ ] 300ml fat-free dressing
- [ ] 500g low-fat mayonnaise
- [ ] 1 packet MAGGI Vegetable Sensations Cajun Wedge Seasoning
- [ ] 2.5 litres MAGGI Real Chicken Stock
- [ ] 1 packet MAGGI Chilli Con Carne Recipe Mix

meat & eggs
- [ ] 600g whiting fillets
- [ ] 1kg pork fillets
- [ ] 500g lean mince OR if using mince for Sherwood Pie instead of TVP (see Seven-day Menu Plan), buy 1.5kg lean mince
- [ ] 1kg lean ham
- [ ] 1 barbecue chicken
- [ ] 500g chicken breast fillets
- [ ] 6 eggs

frozen items
- [ ] 2 litres PETERS Light & Creamy Ice-cream
- [ ] 500g frozen peas
- [ ] 450g frozen spinach

miscellaneous
- [ ] Olive or canola oil spray
- [ ] Olive oil
- [ ] Minced garlic
- [ ] Minced chilli
- [ ] Soy sauce
- [ ] Tomato sauce
- [ ] Black bean sauce
- [ ] MAGGI Sweet Chilli Sauce
- [ ] Small packet caster sugar
- [ ] Small packet brown sugar
- [ ] Vanilla essence
- [ ] Honey
- [ ] Salt and pepper
- [ ] Mixed dried herbs
- [ ] Ground cinnamon and cinnamon stick
- [ ] Saffron threads (optional)
- [ ] Ground nutmeg

seven-day menu plan

Meal	Day 1	Day 2	Day 3	Day 4	Day 5	Day 6	Day 7
Breakfast	Cereal, milk, canned fruit and NESTLÉ All Natural 99% Fat Free Yogurt, Juice	Cereal, milk, canned fruit and NESTLÉ All Natural 99% Fat Free Yogurt, Juice	Baked beans and toast, Juice	Cereal, milk, canned fruit and NESTLÉ All Natural 99% Fat Free Yogurt, Juice	Cereal, milk, canned fruit and NESTLÉ All Natural 99% Fat Free Yogurt, Juice	Canned spaghetti and toast, Juice	Pancakes (packet mix) with fresh fruit and honey Juice
Lunch	Salad sandwiches with ham	Pork in Black Bean Sauce with rice (leftover from Day 1 Dinner)	Salad sandwiches with barbecue chicken	Cream Cheese & Vegie Bagel (page 32)	Toasted sandwiches with Sherwood Pie filling (made with Day 4 Dinner)	Salad sandwiches with tuna and cheese	Ham & Zucchini Risotto (leftover from Day 6 Dinner)
	Fresh fruit	Fresh fruit	Fresh fruit	Fresh fruit	Fresh fruit	Fresh fruit	Fresh fruit
Dinner	Pork in Black Bean Sauce (page 94) (make double quantity for lunch on Day 2)	Tortilla Lasagne (page 48)	Pasta with Chicken & Corn (page 72)	Sherwood Pie (page 56) (make double quantity of filling for lunch on Day 5)* *TVP in recipe can be substituted with lean mince, if preferred	Fish & Chips (page 18)	Ham & Zucchini Risotto (page 74) (make double quantity for lunch on Day 7)	Pizza night – ham and pineapple (use leftover vegetables)
Accompaniments	Rice	Salad	Salad	Salad	Salad	Salad	Salad and bread
Dessert	Steamed Pears (page 100)	Canned fruit with PETERS Light & Creamy Ice-cream	Baked Nectarines with Anzac Crumble (page 24)	Pikelets with PETERS Light & Creamy Ice-cream and banana	Canned fruit with NESTLÉ All Natural 99% Fat Free Yogurt	Creamed Rice with Spiced Apples (page 110)	Fruit salad with PETERS Light & Creamy Ice-cream

quick & easy dinner menu

If a less structured approach to meals suits the group better, then the Quick & Easy Dinner Menu is ideal. Breakfast can be cereal, fruit, yogurt and toast, while lunch can include fresh and toasted sandwiches or leftovers from dinner, and fruit.

This menu has been designed for quick and easy cooking, and includes different cooking styles and flavours that require minimal preparation. The desserts are either from *Survival Around the World* or are simply a combination of items from the supermarket. The recipes are not only quick – they will also use up all the ingredients you've bought and please a crowd.

all you need to do is:

▶ Check that the recipe suggestions suit your needs and make alterations as necessary
▶ If possible, check the availability of cooking equipment in your apartment. You may need to adjust the recipes if important cooking equipment is missing
▶ Pack *Survival Around the World*
▶ Follow the shopping list and buy the ingredients.

Day	Dinner	Dessert
1	Oriental Beef Stirfry (page 120)	Pikelets with PETERS Light & Creamy Ice-cream
2	Spaghetti with Tomato & Chicken Sauce (page 120)	Barney's Blended Juice (page 32)
3	Tuna Pasta (page 120)	Fresh berries (or other seasonal fruit) with yogurt
4	Chilli Beef Burgers (page 120)	Roly Poly – sponge fingers filled with choc hazelnut spread and jam, served with low-fat custard
5	Quick Chicken Pasta (page 121)	Creamed rice with canned passionfruit pulp
6	Pea & Ham Risotto (page 121)	Steamed Pears (page 100)
7	Ham & Tomato Pizza (page 121)	Chopped bananas with PETERS Mango Swirl Ice-cream

shopping list

bread
☐ 8 crusty bread rolls
☐ 1 packet (8) flat breads
☐ 1 packet pikelets

fruit & vegetables
☐ 2 large onions
☐ 1 leek
☐ 300g button mushrooms
☐ 5 tomatoes
☐ 2 carrots
☐ 2 red capsicums
☐ 300g broccoli
☐ Iceberg lettuce
☐ 1 bunch parsley
☐ 8 bananas
☐ 4 large pears
☐ 2 punnets strawberries
☐ 1 punnet blueberries (or other seasonal fruit)

dairy, refrigerated & frozen products
☐ 1 litre pineapple juice
☐ 200g ultra-light sour cream (10% fat)
☐ 2 x 1 litre NESTLÉ All Natural 99% Fat Free Vanilla Yogurt
☐ 1 litre NESTLÉ All Natural 99% Fat Free Fruit Yogurt
☐ 1 litre low-fat custard
☐ 4 individual-sized tubs creamed rice
☐ 250g grated reduced-fat cheese
☐ 125g grated parmesan cheese
☐ 250g low-fat cottage cheese
☐ 1 litre PETERS Light & Creamy Ice-cream
☐ 250g frozen peas
☐ 500g frozen Asian stirfry vegetables

meat
☐ 500g beef strips
☐ 500g lean beef mince
☐ 400g skinless chicken breast fillets
☐ 500g chicken mince
☐ 400g ham

canned & packaged goods
☐ 300g can beetroot
☐ 400g can tuna in spring water/brine
☐ 300g can corn kernels
☐ 3 x 500g jars tomato-based pasta sauce
☐ 500g spaghetti
☐ 500g penne pasta
☐ 500g spiral pasta
☐ 1kg long-grain white rice
☐ 500g arborio rice
☐ 1 litre MAGGI Real Chicken Stock
☐ 375ml can CARNATION Light & Creamy Evaporated Milk
☐ 1 can passionfruit pulp
☐ 1 jar choc hazelnut spread
☐ 200g packet sponge finger biscuits

miscellaneous
☐ olive or canola oil spray
☐ minced garlic
☐ MAGGI Sweet Chilli Sauce
☐ MAGGI Stir Fry Sauce
☐ honey
☐ jam
☐ black pepper
☐ mixed dried herbs
☐ ground nutmeg
☐ ground cinnamon

oriental beef stirfry Serves 4

3 cups long-grain white rice
olive or canola oil spray
500g beef, sliced into strips
1 packet frozen Asian stirfry vegetables
3 tbs MAGGI Stir Fry Sauce

Cook rice according to packet instructions. Spray a non-stick wok or frying pan with oil and cook beef in 2-3 batches over high heat for 2-3 minutes or until browned. Set aside. Reheat wok, add frozen vegetables and 2 tablespoons water and cook until tender crisp. Return beef to pan, add stir-fry sauce and heat through. Serve with rice.

tuna pasta Serves 4

500g penne pasta
250g low-fat cottage cheese
1 cup ultra-light sour cream (10% fat)
400g can tuna in spring water or brine, drained
300g can corn kernels, rinsed and drained
1 red capsicum, finely chopped
freshly ground black pepper

Cook pasta according to packet instructions. Add remaining ingredients and mix to combine. Serve immediately.

spaghetti with tomato & chicken sauce Serves 4

500g spaghetti
olive or canola oil spray
500g chicken mince
500g jar tomato-based pasta sauce
1 red capsicum, chopped
1 cup broccoli florets
1 carrot, peeled and chopped
grated reduced-fat cheese, to serve

Cook pasta according to packet instructions. Meanwhile, spray a wok or large saucepan with oil and cook chicken mince until browned. Add pasta sauce and stir thoroughly. Stir in vegetables and cook for 2-3 minutes. Spoon sauce over spaghetti and serve sprinkled with cheese.

chilli beef burgers Serves 4

500g lean beef mince
1 onion, finely chopped
2 tsp minced garlic
1 tsp mixed dried herbs
2 tbs MAGGI Sweet Chilli Sauce, plus extra, to serve
olive or canola oil spray
8 crusty bread rolls
lettuce leaves, torn
2 tomatoes, sliced
1 carrot, peeled and sliced
beetroot slices

Combine beef mince, onion, garlic, herbs and sweet chilli sauce. Shape into 8 patties and refrigerate, covered, for 15-30 minutes. Spray a non-stick frying pan with oil and cook beef patties over medium heat for 8 minutes. Turn and cook for 5 minutes more. Serve with bread rolls, lettuce, tomato, carrot, beetroot and extra sweet chilli sauce.

quick chicken pasta Serves 4

500g spiral pasta
olive or canola oil spray
400g skinless chicken breast fillets, diced
500g tomato-based pasta sauce
broccoli florets (remainder from Day 2 Dinner)
150g button mushrooms, sliced
grated reduced-fat cheese, to serve

Cook pasta according to packet instructions. Meanwhile, spray a
non-stick pan with oil and cook chicken over medium heat until
cooked through. Stir in pasta sauce and vegetables and simmer
for 5-10 minutes or until just tender. Pour over pasta and toss to
combine. Serve sprinkled with grated cheese.

ham & tomato pizza Serves 4

1 packet (8) flat breads
500g tomato-based pasta sauce
1 onion, finely chopped
150g button mushrooms, sliced
200g ham, chopped
3 tomatoes, sliced
125g grated reduced-fat cheese

Preheat oven to 180°C (350°F). Spread each bread with pasta
sauce and top with onion, mushroom, ham, tomatoes and cheese.
Bake pizzas for 20 minutes, until bases are crisp and golden, and
cheese is melted.

pea & ham risotto Serves 4

olive or canola oil spray
1 leek (white part only), sliced
1 tsp minced garlic
200g ham, chopped
2 cups arborio rice
1 litre MAGGI Real Chicken Stock
375ml CARNATION Light & Creamy Evaporated Milk
1 cup frozen peas
2 tbs chopped fresh parsley
1/3 cup grated parmesan cheese
freshly ground black pepper

Spray a non-stick saucepan with oil and cook leek, garlic and ham
over medium heat for 3-5 minutes or until leek is soft. Add rice and
cook, stirring, for 1 minute or until rice is coated. Add stock and milk
and bring to the boil. Simmer, stirring occasionally, for 20 minutes
or until the rice is soft. Add peas and cook for a further 5 minutes.
Remove from heat and stir through parsley, cheese and pepper.

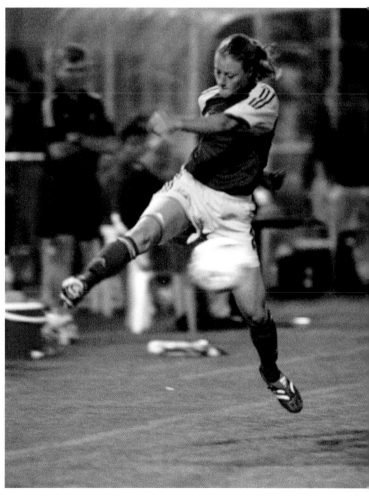

gill foster – soccer player

learning the lingo

Wherever you travel, it helps to have a few basic words and phrases up your sleeve to help you communicate. Most people appreciate it if you make an effort to speak the local language and in some countries it will be essential. The following will help get you started.

Please
French	s'il vous plaît
Greek	parakalo
Italian	per favore
Spanish	por favor
Japanese	dōzo
Mandarin	qǐng
Turkish	lütfen
Vietnamese	làm ơn

I'd like....
French	Je voudrais...
Greek	thathela
Italian	Vorrei...
Spanish	Quisiera...
Japanese	...o kudasai
Mandarin	wǒ yào...
Turkish	...istiyorum
Vietnamese	tôi muốn mua...

Bread
French	du pain
Greek	to psomi
Italian	pane
Spanish	pan
Japanese	pan
Mandarin	miànbāo
Turkish	ekmek
Vietnamese	bánh mì

Fish
French	des poissons
Greek	to psari
Italian	pesci
Spanish	pescado
Japanese	sakana
Mandarin	yú
Turkish	balik
Vietnamese	cá

Vegetables
French	des legumes
Greek	to lachaniko
Italian	verdure
Spanish	verduras
Japanese	yasai
Mandarin	shūcài
Turkish	sebzeler
Vietnamese	rau củ

Water
French	de l'eau
Greek	to nero
Italian	acqua
Spanish	agua
Japanese	mizu
Mandarin	shuǐ
Turkish	su
Vietnamese	nửớc

Thank you
French	merci
Greek	efcharisto
Italian	grazie
Spanish	gracias
Japanese	arigatō gozaimasu
Mandarin	xièxie
Turkish	teşekkür ederim
Vietnamese	cam ơn

Do you have any vegetarian meals?
French	Vous avez des plats végétariens?
Greek	Ehete fagita me lahanika?
Italian	Avete dei piatti vegetariani?
Spanish	Tiene plataos vegetarianos?
Japanese	Bejitarian no ryōri ga arimasu ka?
Mandarin	Ní mēn yǒu méi yǒu zhāi cài?
Turkish	Etsiz yemeğiniz var mı?
Vietnamese	Bạn có những món chay không?

Milk
French	du lait
Greek	to ghala
Italian	latte
Spanish	leche
Japanese	miruku/gyūnyū
Mandarin	niúnǎi
Turkish	süt
Vietnamese	sửa

Meat
French	des viandes
Greek	kreas
Italian	carne
Spanish	carne
Japanese	niku
Mandarin	ròu
Turkish	et
Vietnamese	thịt

Fruit
French	des fruits
Greek	fruto
Italian	frutta
Spanish	fruta
Japanese	kudamono
Mandarin	shuǐguǒ
Turkish	meyve
Vietnamese	trái cây

We enjoyed it/it was delicious etc.
French	C'était très bon, merci.
Greek	Itan katapliktiko, efcharisto.
Italian	Ci è piaciuto, grazie.
Spanish	Nos ha gustado, gracias.
Japanese	Kore wa oishii desu.
Mandarin	Hǎo chī jí le.
Turkish	Hoşumuza gitti, teşekkür ederiz.
Vietnamese	Bà cho ăn ngon quá.

conversion table

conversions

liquid measures

20ml	= 1 tablespoon	
60ml	= $1/4$ cup	= 2 fl oz
80ml	= $1/3$ cup	= $2 3/4$ fl oz
125ml	= $1/2$ cup	= 4 fl oz
250ml	= 1 cup	= 8 fl oz
1 litre	= 4 cups	= 32 fl oz

weight measures

15g	= $1/2$ oz
30g	= 1 oz
250g	= $1/2$ lb
500g	= 1 lb

length measures

2.5mm	= $1/8$ inch
5mm	= $1/4$ inch
1cm	= $1/2$ inch
2cm	= $3/4$ inch
2.5cm	= 1 inch

oven temperatures

	°C	°F	Gas Mark
Very slow	120	250	$1/2$
Slow	150	300	2
Warm (moderately slow)	160	315	2-3
Moderate	180	350	4
Moderately hot	190	375	5
Hot	210	415	6-7
Very hot	230	450	8

glossary

al dente
The texture of cooked pasta when it is ready to eat. Means 'just firm to the bite'.

allspice
A spice made from small sun-dried berries with an aroma of combined cinnamon, cloves and nutmeg. Sold whole or ground.

arborio rice
A variety of short-grain rice usually used to make risotto.

baking
To cook by dry heat in an oven.

bamboo shoots
Young and tender shoots often used to add crispness to Asian soups and stirfries.

basmati rice
White long-grain rice, light in texture with a scented aroma. Used in Indian cooking.

baste
To spoon hot liquid over food as it cooks.

blanch
To place food in boiling water for a short time, then plunge into cold water.

broccolini
A cross between broccoli and the Asian green, gai larn. It has long, thin stems and small florets.

butter beans
Large, flattish, dried white beans that are also known as lima beans.

chat potatoes
Small young potatoes of any variety.

chickpeas
Medium-sized, pale brown, wrinkled peas with a sweet nutty flavour.

choy sum
A Chinese green vegetable with sparse leaves, small yellow flowers and pale green stems. Serve steamed or blanched as a side dish, or in stirfries.

coconut essence
A liquid extracted from coconuts that is used as a flavouring.

couscous
Flour-coated granular semolina which absorbs liquid to become light and fluffy. Popular in Morocco, Tunisia and Algeria.

cracked wheat
Also known as burghul or bulgur, this whole wheat is partially boiled before it is cracked and then dried. It is used in the Middle East as the basis for tabouli.

desiree potatoes
Oval-shaped potatoes with smooth, pink skin and yellow flesh.

dice
To cut into small cubes.

enoki mushrooms
Tiny button mushrooms that grow in clusters on long, slender stems. Use them raw in salads or to garnish soups and cooked dishes.

fish sauce
A flavouring made from small, salted fish, important in Vietnamese and Thai cooking.

garnish
To decorate a dish.

gnocchi
Small Italian dumplings made of choux pastry, semolina flour or potato. They are served with sauce or in soup.

green shallots
Slender white bulbs with straight sides and bright green, hollow tube-like leaves.

grill
To cook using dry heat either under an open grill or on a grill plate.

hummus
A smooth Middle Eastern dip made from pureed chickpeas (see chickpeas), olive oil, lemon juice, garlic and tahini (see tahini).

jalapeño chilli
A dark green chilli that ripens to red and is used in a variety of Mexican dishes and sauces. It is also pickled and canned.

kaffir lime leaves
Also known as makrut, the fresh and aromatic leaves of this lime variety are widely used in Thai and Malaysian cooking.

kidney beans
Medium-sized, kidney-shaped beans that are often used in Mexican cooking.

lemongrass
An aromatic perennial grass native to tropical regions that is used fresh in pastes or to flavour Asian dishes.

marinate
To soak raw foods in an aromatic liquid to increase tenderness and impart flavour.

mirin
A sweet rice wine that is low in alcohol and used in Japanese cooking.

nori
An edible seaweed that is sold in paper-thin strips. It is used to make Japanese sushi rolls or is sliced thinly and sprinkled over soups, noodles or rice.

pickled ginger
Thinly sliced and preserved ginger that is used in Japanese dishes.

poach
To cook food in just enough simmering water or seasoned liquid to cover it, with the lid of the pan off.

puree
To mash and sieve food to make it a smooth consistency.

red wine vinegar
Vinegar obtained from fermented red wine that is used to heighten the flavour of bland foods.

refried beans
Also known as frijoles refritos, these cooked dried beans are mashed to a thick, smooth paste and then fried.

rice paper sheets
Made from rice flour, these paper-thin sheets of dough are dried until stiff. They are used to wrap fresh spring rolls.

rocket
A peppery herb that is often used in salads and sandwiches.

rosewater essence
A natural flavouring that is made from the diluted essence of distilled rose petals. It is often used to flavour Indian and Middle Eastern desserts.

saffron threads
An expensive, pungent, aromatic spice that is obtained from the orange, thread-like stigmas of the purple crocus flower. Used in Asian and Mediterranean dishes.

saute
To fry food briskly using a small amount of oil in a shallow frying pan over moderately high heat, while turning or tossing often.

seasoned rice vinegar
A slightly sweet, mild-tasting vinegar made from fermented rice. It is used in Japanese, Korean and Chinese cooking.

simmer
To keep a liquid just below boiling point so that only small bubbles rise to the surface.

steam
To cook by vapour from boiling water.

sourdough bread
Bread leavened with fermented dough.

spray oil
Olive or canola oil available in a spray can.

sushi rice
Japanese short-grain rice that is used to make sushi.

sweet paprika
A powdered spice that is bright red in colour, made from a mild-tasting red pepper native to Central America.

tahini
A smooth paste made from ground sesame seeds that is used in Greek and Middle Eastern dishes.

textured vegetable protein (TVP)
A fibrous, dehydrated meat alternative usually made by a process that isolates the proteins from soy flour. It is commonly used by vegetarians and is a great substitute for ground beef in tacos, stews and chilli dishes.

tofu
A smooth, custard-like substance made from freshly pressed bean curd. It absorbs the flavours of other ingredients easily and is available soft or firm.

tortilla
A thin, round, unleavened bread made from cornmeal that is used in Mexican dishes as a wrapping.

tzatziki
A cucumber and yogurt salad that is seasoned with crushed garlic, chopped mint, salt and pepper.

wasabi paste
A very hot paste made from the thick, green root of an aquatic plant that is widely used in Japanese dishes.

zest
The coloured, oily outer skins of citrus fruit. Also called the rind.

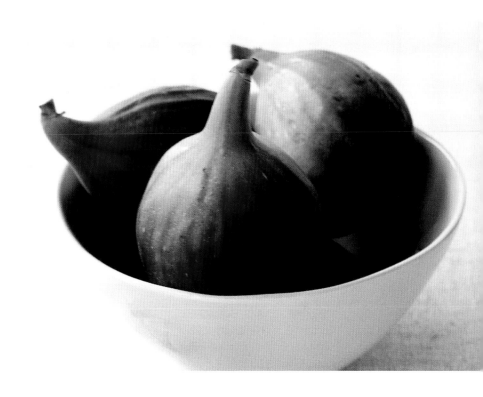

index

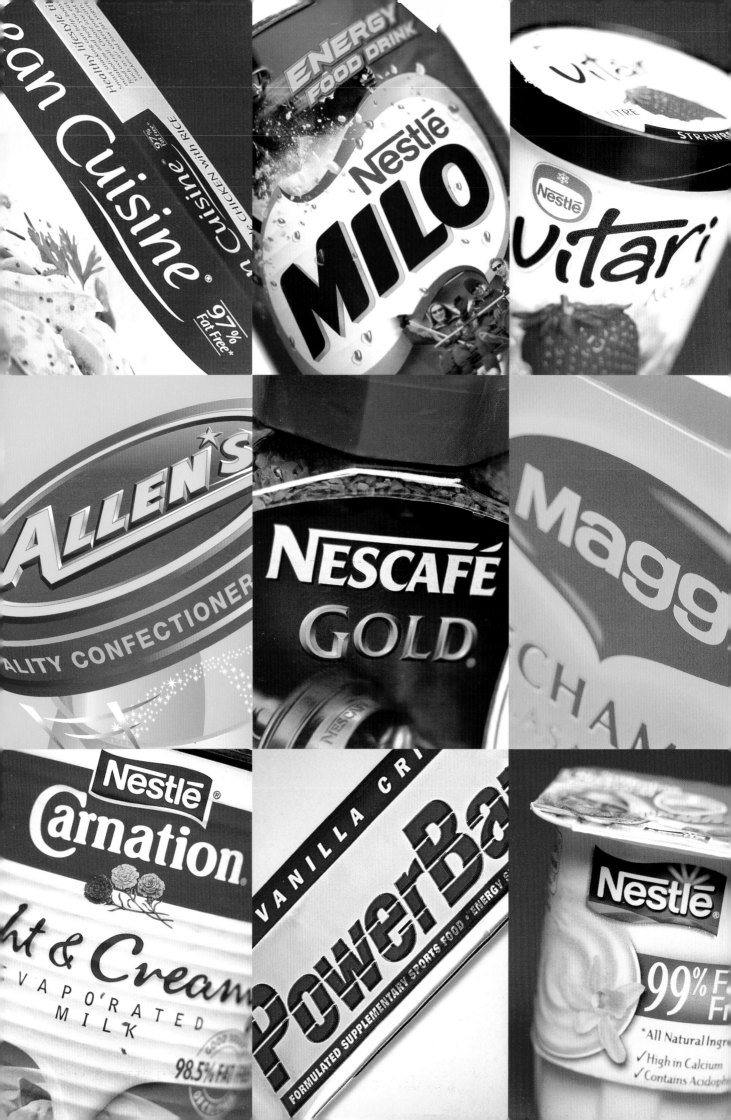